INTERNATIONAL CENTRE FOR MECHANICAL SCIENCES

COURSES AND LECTURES · No. 291

BIOMECHANICS OF ENGINEERING
MODELLING, SIMULATION, CONTROL

EDITED BY
A. MORECKI
WARSAW TECHNICAL UNIVERSITY

Springer-Verlag   Wien GmbH

Le spese di stampa di questo volume sono in parte coperte da contributi
del Consiglio Nazionale delle Ricerche.

This volume contains 85 illustrations.

ISBN 978-3-211-81974-6   ISBN 978-3-7091-2808-4 (eBook)
DOI 10.1007/978-3-7091-2808-4

EDITORIAL NOTE

This book contains the papers presented in the Course on "Biomechanics of Motion" held at the International Centre for Mechanical Sciences, Udine, Italy, 24 through 28 June 1985.

The programme of the course included five working sessions. The papers included in this book appear in the same order as the lectures.

All language corrections and alterations have been reduced to the necessary minimum.

The course of Biomechanics was attended by 26 participants from 12 Countries and six Lecturers from five Countries.

The convenient location of the Center made it possible that a quite large group of scientists could attend. It was also advantageous that all the participants were accommodated in the same premises.

In the editorial note published in the volume "Biomechanics of Motion", which was published by Springer Verlag in 1980 we assumed the constantly increasing significance of biomechanics. The results obtained during the second course confirm this opinion.

A. Morecki

PREFACE

The main purpose of the Course was to present the last scientific results obtained in the field basicly from mathematical and engineering point of view.

The main topics which have been presented and discussed are as follows:

— biomechanics of the upper and lower limbs and their joints: joints replacement. Kinematics of individual joints. Experimental techniques; intersegmental loading.

— mechanical properties of the human muscles involved in a natural motor activity. Electromyographical activity (EMG) and relationship between EMG and biomechanical parameters. Transfer function of natural motor activity.

— data acquisition and reduction in biomechanics. Analysis of human locomotion. Advanced Technologies and Methodologies.

— modelling, mathematical description and measurements of the animal and human body movements. Some selected manipulation and locomotion problems.
Dynamical cooperation of muscle and its control criteria.

— muscle performance. Elastic energy in muscular exercises. Force time curve. Muscle fatigue.

— force and pressure measurements.

— clinical application.

Most of the results, which were presented during the Course were based on the investigation carried on by the invited lecturers.

I hope that this book will be of a strong interest to the readers.

I take the opportunity to express my grateful appreciation to the Authorities of CISM, especially to Prof. G. Bianchi, Secretary General of CISM, for their support of my initiative of the Course "Biomechanics of Motion".

I would like to express my thanks to Prof. G. Longo for cooperation.

A. Morecki

CONTENTS

MODELLING, MATHEMATICAL DESCRIPTION, MEASUREMENTS AND CONTROL OF THE SELECTED ANIMAL AND HUMAN BODY MANIPULATION AND LOCOMOTION MOVEMENTS

A. Morecki
Technical University of Warsaw, Poland

INTRODUCTION

The investigations in the area of Biomechanics of Engineering and Rehabilitation Engineering started at the Technical University of Warsaw in 1961. In the last 24 years several projects were carried out by the interdisciplinary Team of Biomechanics. The list of the main new results obtained in this period of time is as follows:

- mathematical models of isolated muscles included the basic characteristics;

- mathematical models of muscle cooperation in statical and dynamical conditions of the upper extremity of a man;

- statical and dynamical models concerning the problems of biped and fourlegged locomotion;

- design and control of anthropomorphic, bionic and so called "alive" manipulators for supporting or substituting the lost functions of upper human extremities.

These notes will present some latest results obtained in the area of human muscle models included discussion on the influence of some parameters on muscle characteristics. Some remarks on dynamic modelling of relationship between EMG and muscle force will be given. Special attention will be given to the dynamic measurements and control of limbs movement in man, animals and robots. Next, some problems of modelling in athletic movement will be discussed. Manipulation and locomotion problems will be presented on examples of animal locomotion, walking machines and artificial hands. Finally special problems concerning the dynamical cooperation of muscles and mathematical model of a man under vibration will be discussed.

HUMAN AND ANIMALS MUSCLE MODELS

Two muscle models, namely generalized rheological model of isolated muscle and modyfied Hill's two component muscle model will be briefly discussed. In formulating the generalized model we proceed from a common accepted assumption, namely that a force F, which depends on muscle leng l, developed by the muscle during tetanic contraction under constant stimulation, is the sum of the passive component F_p, independent of stimulation, and the active component F_a, dependent of the stimulation value (Fig. 1.1a).

A generalized diagram of the rheological model of the muscle is presented in Fig. 1.1b[1] where the following denotations have been accepted: 1,2,3 - componential units of the model; E_0, E_1, E_2, E_3 - Young modulus val-

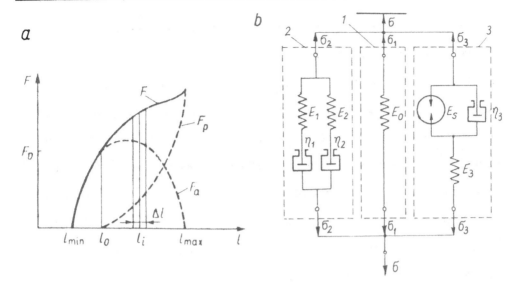

Fig. 1.1. General rheological model of isolated muscle. a – general characteristics of muscle; b – rheological model.

ues of the model's elastic elements in newtons per sq m; E_S – Young modu-

lus describing the force element of the model in newtons per sq m; η_1,

η_2, η_3 – coefficients of viscosity of dumping elements of the model in

newton·secs per sq m; $\sigma_1, \sigma_2, \sigma_3, \sigma$ – stresses for units 1, 2, 3 and for the

whole model respectively in newtons per sq m. With respect to the para-

meters E_0–E_3, E_S, η_1–η_3 and η, it is assumed that they are:

– non-linear functions of muscle length l;

– independent of time (the influence of such parameters as for example

  fatigue is not considered);

– independent of muscle stimulation (the constant stimulation case is

  considered).

    Now we briefly justify why precisely such a pattern of connections

of the componential models has been accepted. A muscle when unstimulated
any passively streched under static conditions behaves like a non-linear
spring with the characteristic $F_p(l)$ (Fig. 1.1a). This state is described by unit 1. The state of an unstimulated muscle under dynamic conditions can be described by unit 2, in which first Maxwell element with
parameters E_1, η_1 describes the so called fast element and the element
with parameters E_2, η_2 the slow element. Unit 3 models the active component of the force developed by the muscle. The research findings of many
authors suggest that the model of the active component should include
what is known as the force contractile component in the considered study
is modelled by the element with the Young modulus E_S, this element describes only the ability of the muscle to develop a force. Moreover, the
viscosity of the muscle when stimulated has been found to change, and in
addition it contains a so called elastic in series component, both having
been allowed for in the model by introducing the elements with parameters
η_3, E_3.

   Depending of the length l of the muscle and its state, particular
combinations of the componential models can be used to describe it behaviour (Table 1.1).

Table 1.1. States of isolated muscle

State of muscles	Muscle length	
	$1 < l_0$	$1 > l_0$
Unstimulated in static conditions	–	1
Unstimulated in dynamic conditions	2	1 + 2
Stimulated in static conditions	3	3
Stimulated in dynamic conditions	2 + 3	1 + 2 + 3

Given below is the set of differential equations describing the model:

$$\sigma_1 = E_0 \varepsilon$$

$$\sigma_2 + \frac{\eta_1}{E_1} + \frac{\eta_2}{E_2} \dot{\sigma}_2 + \frac{\eta_1 \eta_2}{E_1 E_2} \ddot{\sigma}_2 = (\eta_1 + \eta_2)\dot{\varepsilon} + \frac{E_1 + E_2}{E_1 E_2} \eta_1 \eta_2 \ddot{\varepsilon}$$

$$(\sigma_m - \sigma_3)(E_3 + E_S) + \frac{E_3 d(\sigma_m - \sigma_3)}{dt} = \eta_3 E_S \dot{\varepsilon} + E_S E_3 \varepsilon$$

(1.1)

$$\sigma = \sigma_1 + \sigma_2 + \sigma_3$$

where $\sigma_m = E_S \varepsilon^2$ with $\varepsilon_1 = \pm 0,4$.

The first three equations of the system (1.1) describe respectively the units 1, 2 and 3 (Fig. 1.1b); the last one is the notation of parallel connection of the members. Now we proceed to examine more detail the unit 3 which models the active component of the force developed by the muscle under static and dynamic conditions. The parameter E_S is a function of the excitation U and the parameter E_3, a function of the lengthening ε, the muscle stress σ_3 can be given in the form:

$$\sigma_3 = f(U, \varepsilon), \quad E_S = E_S(U)$$

(1.2)

Using the determined static characteristics $\sigma_3(U)$, for different length-ening ε (Fig. 1.2a)[1], we find the parameter E_S in the form:

$$E_S = 6.6\sqrt{U}$$

where the coefficient 6.6 was obtained on experimental data. With a constant excitation U = const, the stress σ_3 (Eq. (1.2)) can be given as:

$$\sigma_3 = E_S f(\varepsilon)$$

(1.3)

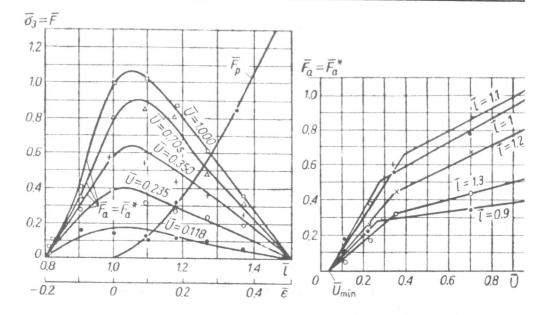

Fig. 1.2. Static characteristics of muscle in frog. a – characteristics $\sigma_3 = f(\varepsilon)$ for different $\bar{U}$; b – characteristics $\bar{F}_a = f(U)$ for different ε, where $\bar{\sigma} = \sigma/\sigma_0$, $\bar{U} = U/U_{max}$, $\bar{\varepsilon} = \varepsilon/\varepsilon_0$.

Next, a function $f(\varepsilon)$ was taken, such as to obtain a conformity between the experimental and simulation responces. The accepted function $f(\varepsilon)$ was in the form of a fourth order polynominal, with weight 1.

Under FLSQFY procedure the problem is solved by the least squares sum method with the use of orthogonal polynominals

$$\sum_{i=1}^{k} w_i \left| P(\varepsilon_i) - \sigma_{3i} \right|^2 = min \qquad (1.4)$$

where $P(\varepsilon_i) = \sum_{i=0}^{k} C_i \varepsilon_i^i$.

Since the approximation by the polynominal was made for $\bar{U} = 1$ hence

$$\sigma_3 = 6.6 P(\varepsilon_i) = 6.6 (C_1 + C_2\varepsilon + C_3\varepsilon^2 + C_4\varepsilon^3 + C_5\varepsilon^4) \qquad (1.5)$$

Values of coefficients C_i are respectively: 0.8732, 1.9932, -14.5921,

3.5061 and 22.5739. Dividing the expression (1.5) by the constant 6.6 we

get the polynominal in the form:

$$f(\varepsilon) = P(\varepsilon_i) = 3.42\varepsilon^4 + 0.53\varepsilon^3 + 2.2\varepsilon^2 + 0.3\varepsilon + 0.13 \qquad (1.6)$$

Using this approximation the response $\sigma_3(\varepsilon)$ for $\bar{U} = 0.118$ was determined

– the approximation error comes to about 10% maximum. A comparison of the

experimental and simulation graphs is given in Fig. 1.3. As seen from the

graphs the coincidence obtained is entirely satisfactory.

A new approach to the human muscle model was given by R.W.A.Baildon

and A.E.Champan[2] in 1983. Hill's (1938) two component muscle model was

used as basis for digital computer simulation of human muscular contrac-

tion by means of an inerative process. The contractile (CC) and series

elastic (SEC) components are lumped components of structures which pro-

duce and transmit torque to the external environment. The authors de-

scribe the CC element in angular terms along four dimensions as a series

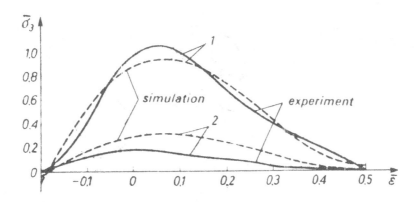

Fig. 1.3. Comparison of experimental and simulation response of muscle
$\bar{\sigma}_3 = f(\bar{\varepsilon})$. 1 – for $\bar{U} = 1$; 2 – for $\bar{U} = 0.118$.

of non-planar torque–angle–angular velocity surfaces stocked on top of
each other, each surface being appropriate to a given level of muscular
activation. The SEC element is described similarly along dimensions of
torque, angular stretch, overall muscle angular displacement and activation. The model allows analysis of many aspects of muscle behaviour as
well as optimization studies. Proposed muscle model is shown in Fig. 1.4.
The CC is a lumped component, consisting of all torque generating structures involved in the analyzed movement. This component is not separated
into individual muscles, fibres or motor units, nor is the rotational
movement translated into the really linear action of the muscles themselves. Similarly the SEC is considered a lumped elastic component, consisting of all elasticity residing in the cross-bridges tendons and any
other elastic structures. These elements are those which transmit torque
from the CC to the external environment.

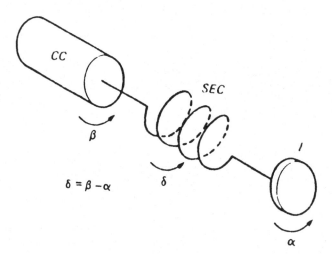

Fig. 1.4. Rotational version of Hill's (1938) muscle model. CC – the
contractile component; SEC – the series elastic component;
I – mass with moment of inertia I; α – limb rotation;
β – CC rotation, the difference is SEC angular stretch, δ.

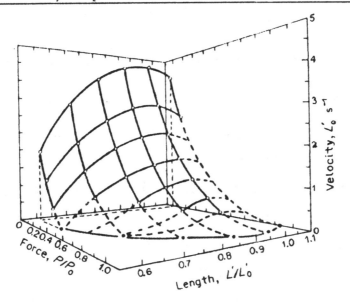

Fig. 1.5. Typical force-length-velocity surface for one activation level.
(Bahler et al., 1968).

Figure 1.5 shows a typical three-dimensional force-length-velocity
surface. Functional properties of the contractile and series elastic components are described by set of equations by Baildon and Chapman[2].

The experimental situation depicted in Fig. 1.4 is that of an inertial load of moment of inertia I being rotated by the limb. The torque
at a given time is determined by

$$T(t) = f(A(t), \alpha(t), \beta(t)), \ N\cdot m \tag{1.7}$$

where A is activation as a fraction (A = 1 in maximal activation); β is
CC velocity $(rad \cdot s^{-1})$ and α is angular muscle displacement. Equation (17)
can be solved for β once all the functions are described. From Fig. 1.4
it also follows that the externally measured torque must be equal to that
transmitted by the SEC, and is thus a function of the parameters de-

scribing the SEC.

Further, the differential equation (1.8) also applies to the system

$$T(t) = I\ddot{a}(t)$$ (1.8)

Not all equations describing the system can be solved simultaneously.
Consequently a stepwise iterative routine was used to provide an approximation as shown in Fig. 1.6. The programme shown in Fig. 1.6 is implemented in the computer language APL on an IBM 4341 computer. When using
linear functions, the system becomes a second order, linear system and
can be evaluated by solving the differential equations describing such a
system. Figure 1.7 shows a comparison of the two solutions. Muscle parameters are those given by Houk (1963) for forearm supination. Moment of
inertia is 0.1 kgm^2. All calculated parameters show very close agreement.

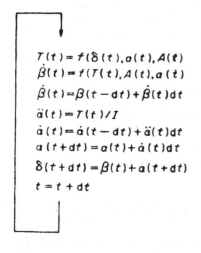

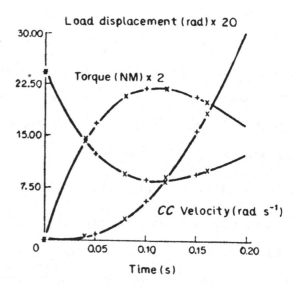

Fig. 1.6. Diagram of iterative
          programme describing
          the proposed muscle
          model.

Fig. 1.7. Torque, angular velocity of
          the CC and load displacement
          all plotted against time.

For the torque time curves, the average error is 0.39%. The new model offered by Baildon and Chapman has several advantages over other models provided in the literature.

An interesting research concerning the influence of muscle temperature, initial length and surface electrical activity on the force-velocity relationship on example of the medial gastrocnemius muscle of the cat was carried on by Petrofsky and Chandler[3]. A special experimental rig was used. Female mougreal cats weighing between 2 and 4 kg were used in these experiments. After special preparation the tendon of the muscle which was to be examined was attached by a steel chain through an LVDT transducer to a variable load (see Fig. 1.8). By moving the lock up and down, the initial position of the muscle before contraction could be adjusted. The temperature of the muscles was maintained at either 28, 32, 35 or 38°C

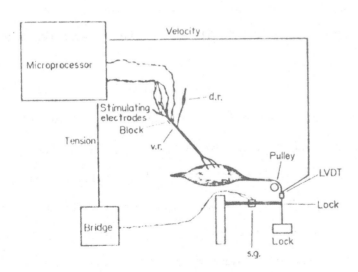

Fig.1.8 Design of the experimental set-up

by   superfusion with liquid paraffin.

The muscles were stimulated sequentially applying a 0.1 ms square wave pulse across 3 pairs of platinum plate electrodes. The frequency of stimulation was set constant at 60 Hz since it has been shown that such a stimulation frequency can fully tetanise these muscles during sequential stimulation (Lind and Petrofsky, 1978; Petrofsky, 1979).

Two series of experiments were conducted on each of four medial gastro-cnemius muscles of the cat. First, following surgery, the maximum iso-metric strength of these muscles was measured by stimulating the muscles with the electric lock left on. The maximum isometric strength was meas-ured at four levels of anodal block which resulted in the muscles develop-ing approximately 25, 50, 75 and 100% of their maximum isometric strength (the isometric strength recorded with all of the motor units recruited). Next, the velocity of shortening was recorded in the unloaded muscles and during contractions against 10 submaximal loads during stimulation at these same levels of anodal block. These experiments were repeated at muscle temperatures of 38, 35, 32 and 28°C. During these contractions, the electrical activity of the muscles was measured by 2 needle electro-des placed on the ends of the muscle. The muscle action potentials were half wave rectified and their rms voltage was then calculated by a digital computer. The computer sampled the electrical activity over 0.2 sec peri-ods through an 8 bit A/D convertor at a sampling rate of 4 kHz. During these experiments, the muscle length was set initially at that length at which the muscle developed its maximum isometric tension.

Next 5 different initial muscle lengths were chosen, these being the lenght at which the muscle developed its greatest isometric

tension with all of the motor units cercuited and, at 0.75,
0,9,1.1 and 1.25 times this length.

The effect of temperature on the force-velocity relationship is
shown in Fig. 1.9 and Fig. 1.10. The force-velocity relationship of the
medial gastrocnemius muscle at a temperature of 38°C is shown in Fig. 1.9
Each point in this figure and in Fig. 1.10 represents the mean of the
results on 4 different muscles contracting at their maximum isometric
strength and at 10 submaximal loads. The average maximum isometric
strength of these muscles with all of the motor units recruited was
3.95 kg, while the isometric strength of these same muscles at the 3 sub-

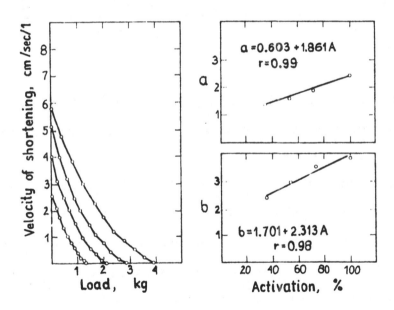

Fig. 1.9. The force-velocity relationship for the medial gastrocnemius
muscle of the cat at 3 levels of submaximal and maximal activation and the resultant Hill   a   and   b   coefficients. Each
point in the figure represents the mean of 4 experiments. The
muscle temperature was kept constant here at 38°C.

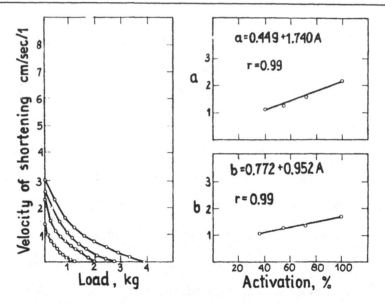

Fig. 1.10. The force-velocity for the medial gastrocniemius muscle of the
          cat at 3 levels of submaximal and maximal activation and the
          resultant Hill "a" and "b" coefficients. Each point in the
          figure represents the mean of 4 experiments. The muscle was
          kept constant here at 28°C.

maximal levels of stimulation averaged 1.38, 2.13 and 2.84 kg. These levels of recruitment then corresponded to 35, 54 and 72% of the maximum
isometric strength of the muscles.

The true relationship between length, temperature and force-velocity
curve was found. The relationship between the Hill "a" and "b" coefficients
of the Hill equation, initial length and temperature of the muscle were
calculated. Figure 1.11 and Fig. 1.12 show some relationship between the
Hill "a" and "b" coefficients and the rms EMG amplitude. The detail discussion can be found in Petrofsky's[3] work.

Independently from deterministic methods, which are used to find the
relationship between EMG and force, in the last years some stochastic mo-

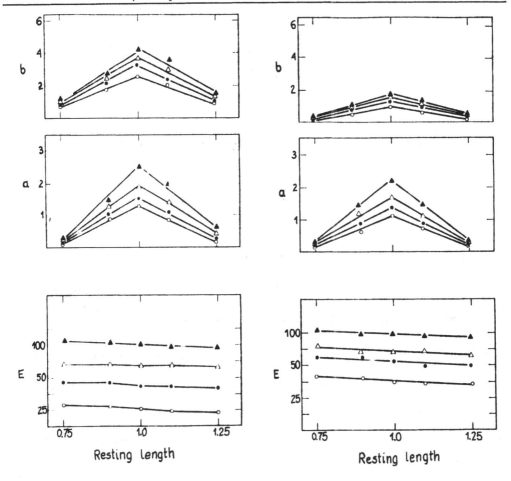

The temperature constant at 38°C   The temperature constant at 28°C

             Fig. 1.11   Fig. 1.12

The relationship between the Hill "a" and "b" coefficients and the rms
EMG amplitude (E) and the length of the muscle (normalized in terms of
the optimum length of the muscle). Each point in these figures represent
the mean of 4 experiments.

dels were proposed. One of the latest model was given by Lago and Jones[4].

Stochastic model is shown in Fig. 1.13, where

$$y(i) = \frac{B(z^{-1})}{A(z^{-1})} s(i) \; ; \quad u(i) = s(i) \cdot d(i) \qquad\qquad (1.9)$$

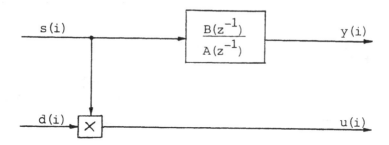

Fig. 1.13. Stochastic model

where i denotes the sampling with respect to time; z^{-1} is the backward

shift operator $(z^{-1}y(i) = y(i-1))$; $A(z^{-1})$ and $B(z^{-1})$ are polynominals in

z^{-1}, of the form $A(z^{-1}) = 1 + \sum\limits_{i=1}^{n} a_i z^{-1}$ and $B(z^{-1}) = b_0 + \sum\limits_{i=1}^{n} b_i z^{-1}$ re-

spectively; s(i) is nonnegative; d(i) is a nongegative stationary colour-

de random sequence statistically independent of s(i) with E d(i) = 1;

y(i) is the noise-free output of a linear dynamical system driven by the

unmeasurable input signal s(i); u(i) is measurable input described by s(i)

modulated by d(i).

Experiments were carried out on normal lightly muscled subjects

using isometric contractions of the right deltoid. The EMGs were amplified

band pass-filtered and, together with the force signal, recorded on a FM

stoperecorder for further processing. A parametric description of the re-

lationship between the rectified EMG and the force can easily be derived

from the Lago model in form

$$EMG(i)| = C_i \cdot \rho(i)d(i) ; \qquad f(i) = \frac{C_2 B(z^{-1})}{A(z^{-1})\rho_i} \qquad (1.10)$$

where $C_1 = E||s(i)||$; $d(i) = C^{-1}|s(i)|$, a coloured random sequence sta-
tistically independent of $\rho(i)$; $\rho(i)$ is the unmeasurable intensity function of the generating point process underlying both the EMG and the force.

More information on development of the instrumental variables method, which is useful when the noise is amplitude modulated by the input
signal can be found in Lago and Jones[4] work.

DYNAMIC AND CONTROL OF LIMBS MOVEMENTS

Certain limb movements elicited by visual stimuli are currently
assumed to be controlled by "programs" that generate instructions appropriate for activating the spinal motoneurons. Our knowledge about the
organization and the characteristics of these programs is relatively low,
it is not yet clear which aspects of movements are controlled by these
programs.

We will briefly discuss some results obtained by Polit and Bizzi[5]
(1978) in processes controlling arm movements in monkeys. Three adult
rhesus monkeys were trained in pointing task. The monkeys sat in a pri-
mate chair with right forearm fastened to an apparatus that permitted
flexion and extension of the forearm about the elbow in the horizontal
plane. The pointing task required that the monkey position its limbs in
front of a small target light. The monkeys were trained to point to
whichever light was on and to hold the arm at that position for about
sec. The experiments were conducted in a dark room to restrict visual
eyes to the target. The arm was either loaded or unloaded. Some hypotheses were assumed and tested, namely that efferent proprioceptive infor-

mation changed the oryginal motor command or that the motor programme underlying arm movement specifies, through the selection of a new set of length-tension curves, and equilibrium point between agonist and antago-nists that correctly positions the arm in relation to the visual target. To investigate the applicability of this hypothesis to arm movements we restored the monkey's performance after it had undergone a bilaterale dorsal rhizotomy from the first cervical through the third thoracic root. No significiant differences were found in the three monkeys both before and after deafferentation (Fig. 2.1).

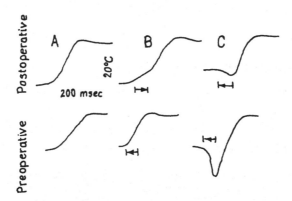

Fig. 2.1. (Preoperative) Visually elicited arm movements made by an in-
        tact monkey during pointing task. (A) Normal, unloaded move-
        ment. (B) Arm movement with which the torque motor moved the
        limb toward the target zone. (C) An instance in which the tor-
        que motor had displaced the forearm away from the target. In
        both (B) and (C), the forearm reached the correct final position.
        Timing and duration of the load application are indicated by
        arrows. (Postoperative) Visually evoked arm movement made by
        the same monkey after bilateral dorsal rhizotomy from the
        second cervical to the third thoracic vertebrae in response to
        visual targets but without sight of its arm. In (B) a transient
        torque displaced the arm toward the target zone, whereas in (C)
        the load displaced it away from the target zone. The target
        light was on during actual pointing. In both preoperative and
        postoperative conditions, the initial forearm position was
        different from trial to trial[5].

These results thus suggest that what is being programmed is an intended
equilibrium point resulting from the interaction of agonist and antagonist muscles. Polit and Bizzi concluded, based on observations that no
radical changes in motor programming during the days immediately following the rhizotomy, that in both in fact and deafferented monkey's,
visually evoked arm movements seem to depend at least in part, upon a
process that specifies final position. On the other words visually evoked
movements may results in part from commands that shift the equilibrium
point between agonist and antagonist muscles.

In the second part of this chapter we will describe some results
obtained in:

- acquisition and analysis of electromyographic data associated with dynamic movements of the arm (Johnson, Lynn, Gandy, Reed, Miller[6], 1980);
- spatial control of arm movements (Morosso[7], 1981);
- organization of visual spatial functions in human cortex; evidence from
  electrical stimulation (Freed, Mateer, Ojemann, Wonhs, Fedio[8], 1982);
- central nervous control of arm movement in stroke patients (Hammond,
  Miller, Robertson[9], 1982).

We will shortly describe the main results obtained during the investigations performed by mentioned above teams in the last years.

A standarized movement task has been developed for an investigation
of normal patterns of electromyographic (EMG) activity. The subject is
required to turn a cranked wheel with his arm which is supported horizon-
tally in front of him (Fig. 2.2). The movements were standarized by posi-
tioning the subject using anatomical landmasks and is defined by the
angle of the wheel.The performed measurements of EMG signals

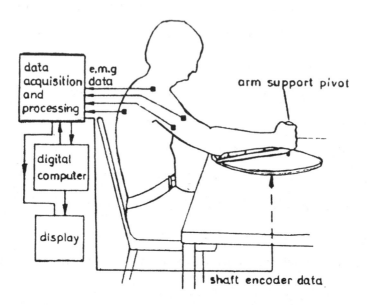

Fig. 2.2. Subject turning cranked wheel.

from a group
of arm and trunk muscles (20 normal subjects), shows that characteristic
patterns of EMG activity in relation to the position of the wheel can be
defined. In Fig. 2.3 a typical normal pattern of muscle activities is
shown. From performed experiments is clear that a simple movement task
can give reliable and repeatable patterns of EMG activity.

Another interesting research on spatial control of arm movements
was carried out by Morosso[7]. Human subjects were instructed to point one
hand to different visual targets which were randomly sequenced, using a
paradigm which allowed two degrees of freedom (shoulder, elbow). The time
course of the hand trajectory and the joint angular curves were observed.
The hypothesis was formulated that the control command for these movements
is formulated in terms of spatial trajectories of the hand in space.

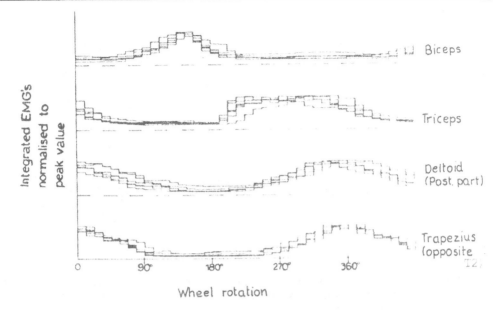

Fig. 2.3. Six patterns for a single normal subject obtained in separate
          recording sessions over a period of three weeks.

Movements of the arm can be described either in terms of spatial trajectories of the hand or of angular curves of the joints. It is thus
important to determine whether the motor commands are centrally represented in terms of joints angles or of spatial trajectories. In order to
answer this question, it is possible to observe different movements
which correspond to the same motor task and to look for common features
among the different movements.

The experimental paradigm was chosen in such a way as to simplify
the problem as much as possible; only two degrees of freedom were allowed
and the influence of gravity was kept constant by working in the horizontal plane. In this way, movements of the arm were reduced to flexion-extension of the elbow and flexion-extension of the shoulder (Fig. 2.4).

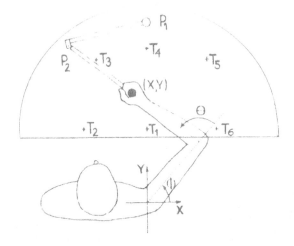
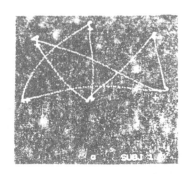

Fig. 2.4. Experimental setup for the study   Fig. 2.5. Spatial trajectory
          of reaching movements in the   of the hand.
          horizontal plane.

Trunk movements were presented by appropriate strapping. Six adults participated as subjects in the experiments during which the six targets
were activated according to a sequence (the activation sequence of the
targets included 30 targets, it was randomized in space and in time, with
an average activation interval of 3 sec), which was repeated five times,
with a small rest time between trials. An example of the experiments is
presented in Fig. 2.5. In sum, the observations above may be summized by
saying that the common features among the different reaching movements
are the single packed shape of the hand tangential velocity and the shape
of the hand trajectory. As a consequence Morosso concludes, that spatial
control hypothesis may be consider what means that the central commands
which underlie the observed movements are more likely to specify the
trajectory of the hand than the motion of the joints.

Bernstein (1935) formulated the hypothesis that there exist in the higher levels of the CNS projections of space and not projections of joints and muscles. The same kind of problem is being in the robotic field. Even if most industrial robots presently used are controlled according to joint--oriented schemes, the need of task-oriented control systems is favoring the emergence of concepts of "spatial control" (Nevis and Whitney, 1973, Paul, 1979). Since the subjects in Morosso's study tended spontaneously to produce straight hand path, Fried and others[8] investigated the movements strategies used by subjects who had been instructed to use curved hand path to reach a target. Movements of the right arm were studied in 15 normal, right-handed subjects (9 women and 6 men), who ranged in age from 20 to 38 years. Each subject gave informed consent to the experimental procedures. The experimental apparatus is illustrated in Fig. 2.6. The subject was seated and grasped the vertical handle of a hand-position transducer. An example is shown in Fig. 2.7. Three experiments were con-

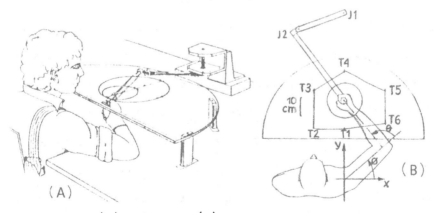

Fig.2.6.Oblique(A) and plan(B)views of a seated subject
     grasping the handle of the hand-position transducer.

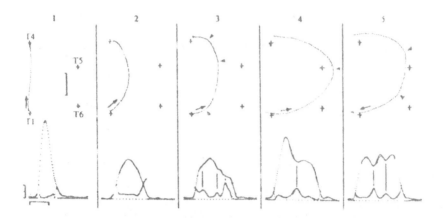

Fig. 2.7. Five movements recorded form the same object with no guide pre-
        sent. In 1, the subject was told to move hand to the target,
        in 2 to 5, to use a curved path to reach the target.

ducted. In the first, the subject was instructed to move his hand to the

target by way to curved path; in the second, he was told to move his hand

to the target along straight of curved guide paths; and in the third, he

moved his hand around an obstacle to reach the target. Two remarkable

findings were obtained. The first is as follows: when the subjects were

given no instruction regarding trajectory but were told to move their

hand deliberately to a target, the paths have been noted both in man

(Morosso, 1981) and in monkey (Gilman, 1976). This tendency presents even

when subjects were told to produce curved paths. The second finding re-

gards the irregular character of the speed profiles associated with curved

trajectories. It is interesting to note that a given task entails similar

problems of control for both artificial and biological systems. In pro-

ducing arm trajectories each system must have a mechanism for associating

hand paths and joint torques. In general, the task of reaching for an object in space with a man-made multijoint system requires that the path

of the terminal joint of the manipulator be specified, usually in Carte-

sian coordinates. The problem of performing a transformation from Carte-

sian coordinates to joint-coordinates (inverse kinematics) and then ob-

taining the required joint torques (inverse kinematics) has been ap-

proached in two ways, one based on computational procedures (that is

rest-time processing) and the other on lock-up tables (that is memory).

Recently (Luk, 1980; Hollerbach, 1980) some of the terms of the equation

of motion are precomputed and stored on memory, and the others are com-

puted on a real-time basis.

In order to develop a biological perspective on trajectory formation

in vertebrates three possible explanations were considered, namely

- the trajectory characteristics may arise from the intrinsic properties

  of the muscles and their geometrical arrangements;

- that for curved paths, the control system generates a series of force

  vectors acting at the hand, the orientation of each vector roughly

  paralleling the intended curved trajectory;

- the third possible explanation of the curvature and speed features of

  curved movements emphases central control factors rather than the geo-

  metric and physical properties of the arm have the CNS would plan a

  movement.

The last problem presented in this chapter concerns some experimen-

tal results obtained during measurements of arm movements of normal sub-

jects and hemiplegic patients. It is commonly accepted that the disorder

of voluntary movement of the arm observed in stroke patients results from interruption of cortifugal nerve fibres, since most lesions occur in the celebral hemisphere or internal capsula (Hammond, Miller, Robertson[9], 1982). In that case the spinal motor centres controlling arm movements are partly deprived morphologically and/or functionally of projections from various supraspinal centres. During the performed experiments the subject sits in an anatomically standarized position at the table in which the cranked weel is set (see Fig. 2.8). He was required to turn the

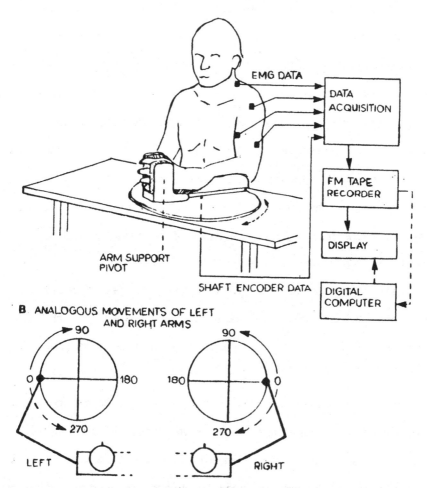

Fig. 2.8 A cranked wheel task

cranked wheel a number of revolutions in each direction with each arm.

The normal subject and 10 stroke patients were tested. The EMG patterns

for analogous arm movements of normal subjects are similar on right and

left sides (Fig. 2.9). In unaffected arm of stroke patients the EMG pat-

terns are comparable to those of normal subjects and serve of individual

controls of the affected arm (Fig. 2.10). The EMG patterns obtained du-

ring the task from the affected arms of stroke patients differed in

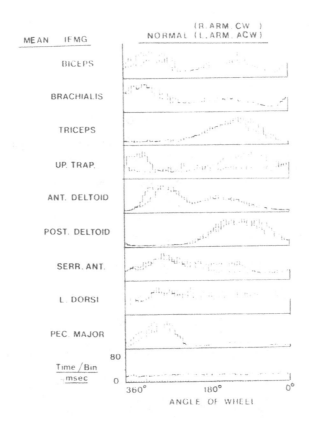

Fig. 2.9. Analogous mirror image movements. Overplot of patterns in the
          right arm clockwise (CW) and left arm anticlockwise (ACW)
          directions in same normal subject to show equivalence of these
          mirror image movements.

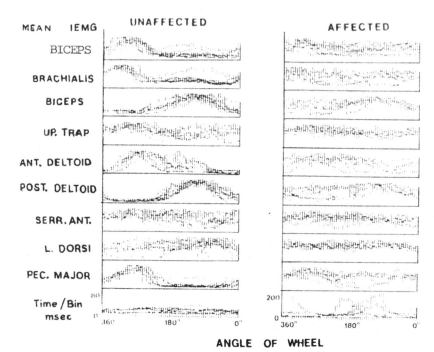

Fig. 2.10. Mean integrated EMGs (IEMG) and time per wheel position bin
versus wheel position. Overplots of averages obtained during
10-20 revolutions of the wheel in 8 hemiplegic stroke patients
performing functionally analogous arm movements.

several respects from those of their unaffected arms and from those of

normal subjects. In particular, transitions between flexion and extension

were prolonged, and abnormal co-contraction of antagonist muscles occured.

MODELLING IN ATHLETIC MOVEMENT

The science of biomechanics of sport and physical education has been

developed rapidly during the last decade. Central to this progress has

been the development of sophisticated research and instrumentation sys-

tems (Nelson[36], 1978). We will shortly discuss following problems:

- dynamic of the pole vault;

- optimal running of skis in downhill;

- simulation of modified human airborne movements;

- a model for the calculation of mechanical power during distance running;

- biomechanics of optimal flight in ski-jumping;

- dynamic and static lifting.

The main goal of this chapter is to present the possibilities of mathematical modelling of very complicated movements of a man during different sport activities. Based on rather simple mechanical models it is possible to investigate different aspects of movement.

A comprehensive study in dynamic modelling of the pole vault was carried out in Poland by a research group conducted by J.Morawski[10]. A simple model of the vaulter-pole system was used for the investigations. The following simplifying assumptions were accepted:

- the movement of the vaulter is treated as plane, taking place in vertical plane at right angle to the bar axis;

- the vaulter is treated as a mass reduced to a single point coinciding with the centre of the body;

- the mass of thepole is neglected;

- the elastic properties of the pole are simulated by an nonlinear element[36].

The model of the system accepted for the analysis is shown in Fig. 3.1.

The horizontal and vertical components of the force occuring in the pole can be expressed in the form:

$$R_x = R \frac{x}{\sqrt{x^2 + y^2}} \tag{3.1}$$

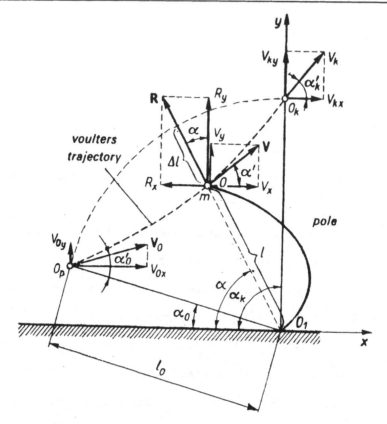

Fig. 3.1. Simple model of pole vault.

$$R_y = R \frac{y}{\sqrt{x^2 + y^2}} \tag{3.2}$$

where R is a force being a function of pole flexion Δl. The flexion Δl can be expressed in the form:

$$\Delta l = l_0 - \sqrt{x^2 + y^2} \tag{3.3}$$

where l_0 is the length of unflexed pole (the distance, measured along the pole, between the grip of the pole and its end placed in the hollow of the box). For simplification, we accept that the grip is a point corresponding to the vaulter's upper hand. The movement equations have been

given a convenient form for analog modelling

$$m\ddot{x} - R \frac{x}{\sqrt{x^2 + y^2}} = 0$$

$$m\ddot{y} - R \frac{y}{\sqrt{x^2 + y^2}} + mg = 0$$

(3.4)

The equations (3.4) describe the movement of the vaulter treated as a

particle both in the phase in which the vaulter is "connected the pole"

and in the airborne phase as he lets it go. The equations of the analysed

process are useful for modelling and the model represents a system with

two degrees of freedom.

To solve the equations a Solarton MS7-2 computer was used. the tra-

jectories of the centre of mass of the vaulter as shown in Fig. 3.2 are

obtained by model tests. To illustrate the time function of the vault the

trajectories of the vaulter have been plotted as dashed lines, where O_p

is initial point of the trajectories; h_a is terminal hight for the tra-

jectory a, as against the trajectory b, where only section h_b was recog-

nized as such. Trajectory c corresponds to an unsuccessful jump, in which

the competitor has been thrown back to by the pole. Example test results

are presented in Fig. 3.3. The optimum curse of the vault is obtained for

an initial horizontal velocity of about 9.05 ms^{-1}. The influence of the

vaulter's mass for constant parameters of the pole is illustrated in

Fig. 3.4. Further step in modelling of the pole vault was done by Hub-

bord[11] (1980). More realistic system model was proposed. A schematic

diagram of the complete model is given in Fig. 3.5.

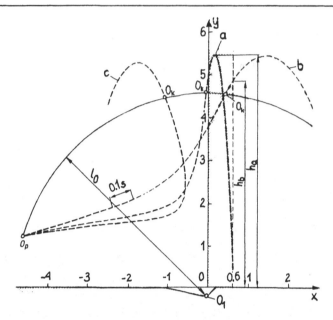

Fig. 3.2. General diagram of solution.

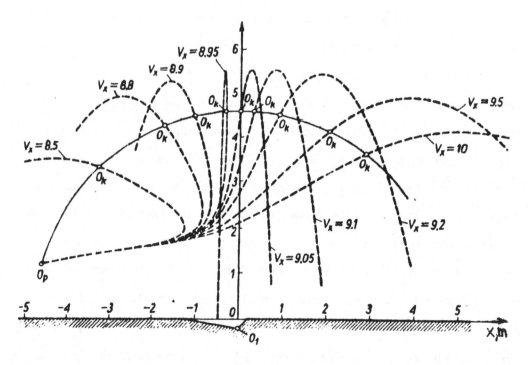

Fig. 3.3 Trajectories of jumper's centre of mass in pole valut for diff v_x

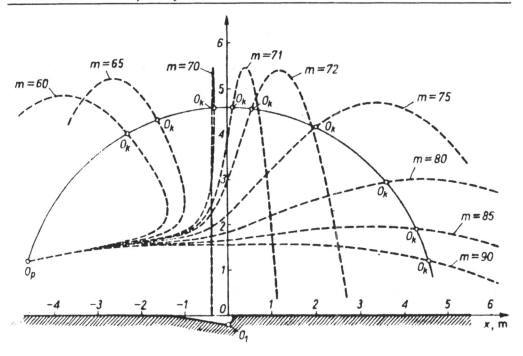

Fig. 3.4. Trajectories of jumper's centre of mass in pole vault for different body weight values m (kg).

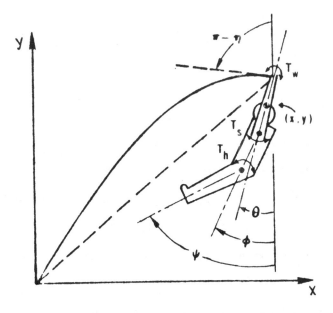

Fig. 3.5. Schematic diagram of vaulter pole system.

The five degrees of freedom (yielding a system of 10 ordinary first-order differential equations) are the position coordinates (x,y) of the center of mass (c.m.) of the arms, and the three orientations of the rigid body segments (θ,ϕ,ψ). Three rigid bodies are hinged at the hip, shoulder and wrist and the voluntary control torques (T_w,T_s,T_h) are exerted by the vaulter at three points. The motion of the vaulter-pole system will be assumed to take entirely in the saggital plane of the vaulter, which remains perpendicular to end constains the center of the cross bar. A simple first order muscle dynamic model was assumed. Bond graphs are chosen to formulate the system model equations. The equations can be presented in a form:

$$A(\bar{x})\dot{\bar{x}} = D(\bar{x})\bar{x} + G(\bar{x})\bar{u} + \bar{h}(\bar{x}) \qquad (3.5)$$

where the state vector

$$\bar{x} = \left[x,y,\theta,\phi,\psi,\ \dot{x},\dot{y},\dot{\theta},\dot{\phi},\dot{\psi},T_w,T_s,T_h\right]^T \qquad (3.6)$$

and the control vector

$$\bar{u} = \left[T_w,T_s,T_h\right]^T \qquad (3.7)$$

The coefficient matrices A, D and G are functions of the state vector and the vector $\bar{h}(\bar{x})$ includes the effects of gravity. The equations can be integrated numerically to obtain the state vector $\bar{x}$ as a function of time. The trajectories of the c.m. of the vaulter and of the handhold are shown in Fig. 3.6. The position and shape of the pole are shown at the time t = 0.54 s of minimum chard length (0.52 L). Figure 3.7 shows the angles θ,ϕ,ψ versus time for the same vault. By using the two described models, it should be possible to calculate the optimal control torques given a particular set of initial conditions and answer many other questions.

The next problem is concerned with optimal running of skis in downhill. The ski-turn with the skis run close and parallel to each other is according to Morawski[12] a typical example of the inverted "pendulum" with its fulcrum being fluidly displaced (Fig. 3.8a). The control of the transverse movement of the skier's body plays an important part here. To simplify the analysis it is assumed that the skier's is processing on a flat horizontal surface or on a slightly inclined shape. Figure 3.8b shows a skier performing a ski-turn. The results of analysis can be found in some works[12, 36]. Further development in this area was done by Remizov[13] who

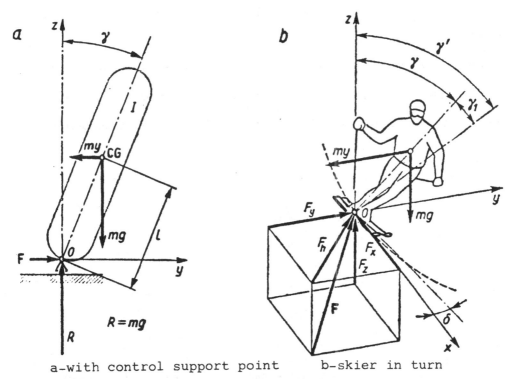

a-with control support point   b-skier in turn

Fig. 3.8 Inverted pendulum model

consider a planar model of a skier performing downhill (that is straight

running, traverse, passage of bump, gulley, etc.) in vertical plane in

order to minimize the time of his descent. Figure 3.9 shows force diagram.

The force exerted on the skier during the shuss are the frictional force

F, air resistance Q, lifting force Y, weight mg and normal reaction N.

The displacement of the center of gravity of the skier-skis system in a

fixed position down the even slope may be described then by the differen-

tial equation of the second order with constant coefficients,

$$\frac{dv}{dt} = - bv^2 + a , \qquad v = \frac{dx}{dt} , \tag{3.8}$$

where v is velocity; x is coordinate (along the full line); b = $1/2 m_\rho SC_x$;

m is mass of the system; a = g(sinα - kcosα) is angle of slope; k is co-

efficient of friction; t is time.

It exist the solution of equation (3.8) in quadrature formula; therefore

it is possible to perform a full investigation of kinematics of a racer

during his motion along the fall line of fixed slope. The calculations

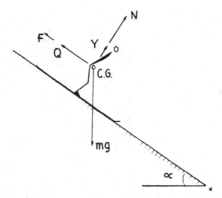

Fig.3.9 Force diagram of a skier on the slope

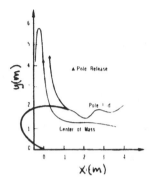

Fig.3.6 Trajectories of the vaulter center of mass and pole
grip point during nominal vault.

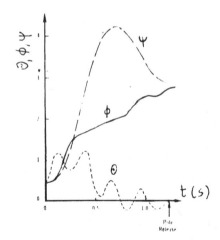

Fig.3.7. Vaulter body segmental orientations (θ, ϕ, ψ)
vs time during nominal vault.

were performed for "Kilometro Lanciato" race. Remizov computed the equa-

tion (3.8) in order to reconstruct the record run (174.717 km·h^{-1}) of

the Italian Luigi di Marco in 1964 (his weight was known). By k=0.02

frontal air resitance coefficient $\mu = \frac{1}{2}SC_x\rho = 0.013$ kgs^{-2}m^{-2}. Remizov's

model reached an average speed 174.5$\pm$0.9, which gives a satisfactory

agreement with experiments in wind tunnel (Gorlin, 1972). Some other

problems like the fastest shuss with speed limitation, optimal up-traken,

optimal running trajectory synthesis were solved. To solve the problem

of the optimal ski descent with the speed limitation, the basic theorem

of the optimal control theory "Pontriagin maximum principle" has been

applied. Figure 3.10 shows some results obtained during these investiga-

tions.

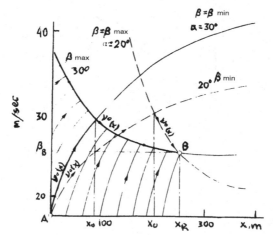

Fig.3.10 Family of optimal phase trajectories of a shuss on
the 10° slope with the finish at point B(x_B = 43 m;
v_B 14.6 m/s)

We will present two models concerning the force distribution aerodynamic moments in ski-jumping. In Fig. 3.11 the assumed reference system, system of forces and moments affected the ski-jumper during flight
suggested by J.Maryniak[14] is shown. To investigate the dynamic properties
in motion it is necessary to know the aerodynamic coefficients like:
carrying capacity C_z, inclining moment C_m, side force C_y and deviating
moment C_u. Aerodynamic coefficients have been experimentally fixed for
several human figures on skis. In order to carry out a comparison on the
aerodynamic properties of particular figures, an aerodynamic perfection
had been introduced such as for flying objects

$$k = \frac{C_z}{C_x} ,$$

(3.9)

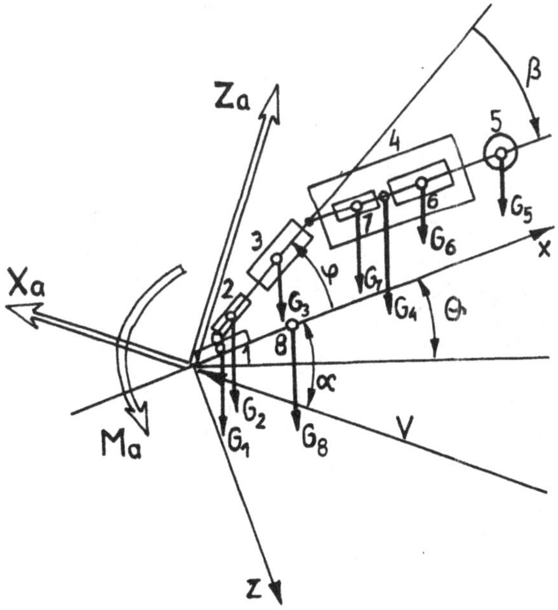

Fig. 3.11. The assumed reference system and system of forces and moments
effecting the ski-jumper during flight.

where k is relation of the carrying capacity coefficient C_z to the coef-

ficient of resitance C_x (Fig. 3.12). Remizov[15] studied the flight in a

vertical plane of a ski-jumper after take-off with the purpose of maxi-

mizing flight distance. To solve the problem of optimal flight (how a

jumper must change his angle of attack to obtain the longest jump) the

basic theorem of the optimal control theory - Potriangin's maximum prin-

ciple - was applied. The calculations were based on data from wind tunnel

experiments. The flight length in ski-jumping depends not only on the

tangential and normal velocity components (due, respectively, to runway

speed and push-off thrust) but is substantially influenced by the skier's

posture in the air and by the change of this orientation to the flow of

air (angle of attack) during the flight (Komi, 1974; Maryniak, 1975).

Figure 3.13 shows the reference system and some kinematic and dynamic

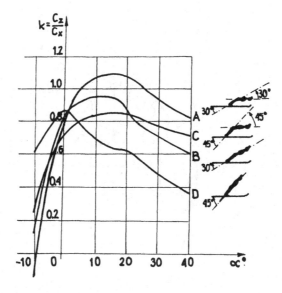

Fig. 3.12. Aerodynamic perfection of a ski-jumper k in the angle of
attack function α for different configurations of skis and
body A, B, C and D.

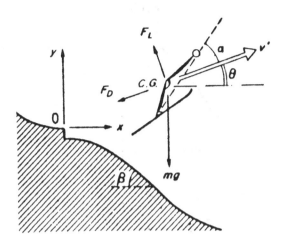

Fig. 3.13. Profile contour of a jumping hill and the corresponding co-
          ordinate system. Forces affecting the skier in the air, flight
          angles.

parameters assumed for analysis. The problem of optimal control consists

in determining the control $\alpha(t')$ which could lead to the achievement of a

maximal jump length measured according to the compatition rules from the

edge of the take-off ramp (point 0). The largest jump is equivalent to

the achievement of the maximum value of abscissa $x(T')$ at the instant of

landing T'. A problem formulated like that is the rotational problem with

a free right bound and time unfixed (Pontriagin et al., 1961) which re-

quires maximizing the function

$$J = x(T') \tag{3.10}$$

The solution of the problem of optimal control of a flight of a ski-jump-

er was found[15]. The equations were numerically solved using the method of

consecutive approach (Krylov et al., 1972). Figure 3.14 shows the pattern

of optimal change in the angle of attack affording the maximal flight

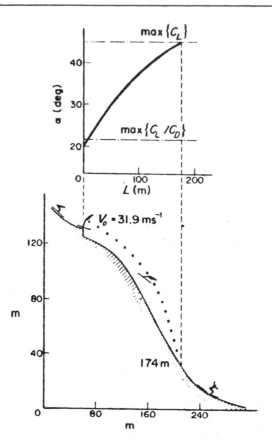

Fig. 3.14. Optimal flight path on the Planica jumping hill and corresponding optimal angle of attack.

length of 174 m with initial speed 31.9 ms^{-1}.

A method of simulation of modified human airborne movements was proposed by Dapena[16] in 1981. In the method an airborne activity is filmed
with two high-speed motion picture cameras. The films are subsequently
analysed to calculate time-dependent three dimensional coordinates of
21 body landmarks. The method was divided into two stages: analysis of
the actual motion of the subject and generation of the simulated motion

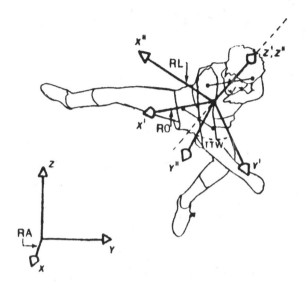

Fig. 3.15. RA, RO and RL reference frames.

of the subject. A series of Fosburg-flop style high jumps and diverse

trampolining stunts were filmed. The reference frames are shown in Fig.

3.15. The body was assumed to be composed of 15 rigid segments. The data

were taken from Dempster's (1955) cadarer data. The generation of simu-

lated motion (stage 2) was carried out by a computer programme. There are

some limitations of the method concerning simulation procedure and point

torques values.

An interesting procedure for determining angular positional data

relative to the rotational axes of the human body was proposed by Gervais

and Marino[17]. A simple computational procedure for determining angular

displacement-time histories of human motion from three-dimensional cine

data was given. This method based on algebraic transformations of coordi-

nates and coordinate axes. Figures 3.16 and 3.17 show the relative angular

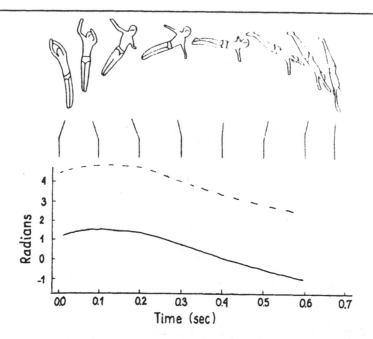

Fig. 3.16. Upper and lower body center of mass around the pith axis.

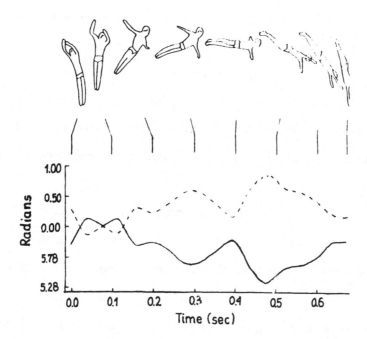

Fig. 3.17 Upper and Lower body center of mass around the roll axis

positional-time data obtained for the flight phase of the arabian dive roll.

In this section we will shortly discuss two models, namely: for static lifting : relationship of loads on the spine and the knee and dynamic biomechanical evaluation of lifting maximum acceptable loads.

In the first case an experimental study based on a trigonometric, anthropometric model was conducted on thirty five healthy subjects to determine the relationship between knee and back forces during symmetric saggital plane lifting. Total joint reaction forces for the knee and the back, along with their compressive and shear components, were calculated for each subject, as a function of the knee, back and ankle angles (Bejjani, Gross and Pugh[18]). A simple, two-dimensional static model was used (Fig. 3.18). The model represents the projection in a saggital plane of the mechanical axes of the spine and the dominant upper and lower limbs of an individual. For the analysis a free-body diagram was used (Fig. 3.19). All data were analyzed statistically. Two major studies were performed: a comparison between back and knee forces for each subject and a comparison between males and females. A very high inverse correlation was found between knee and back forces for all subjects.

Other important correlations were found, too. It was shown, in particular, that for lifting a load of 0.2 m height and representing 10% of total body weight, one must bend both back (about 60%) and knees (about 90%) in order to minimize the average force. Figure 3.10 shows some results obtained during the experiments.

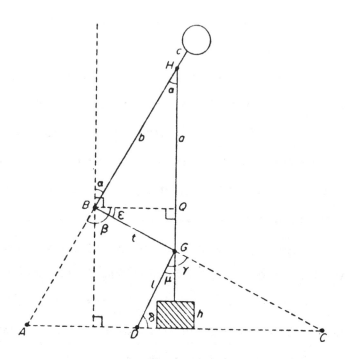

Fig. 3.18. Trigonometric and anthropometric model of lifting. α – back
flexion angle; β – hip flexion angle; γ – knee flexion angle;
ε – angle between thigh and horizontal; δ – angle between foot
and leg; μ – angle between vertical and leg; B – center of
rotation of the hip; G – center of rotation of the knee;
a – distance between acromion and 3rd PIP joint; b – distance
between T1 and 3rd coccygeal vertebra; c – distance between
T1 and vertex; t – distance between greater trochanter and
lateral condyle; 1 – distance between lateral femoral condyle
and heel; h – height of the load.

The general purpose of Freivalds and others[19] contribution is to de-

scribe the development of a methodology for analyzing the amount of stress

imposed on a person's muscular-skeletal system, especially to low back,

during infrequent manual materials handling (MMH) tasks. More specifical-

ly there are three objectivities namely: to detail the implementation of

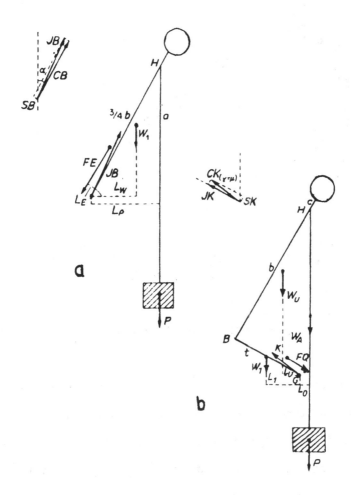

Fig. 3.19. Free body diagram. a) FE – erector spinae force; LE – lever arm of the erector spinae; W_1 – weight of the head, torso and arms; L_W – lever arm of W_1; P – weight of the load; L_p – lever arm of the load; JB – joint reaction force; CB – compression force; SB – shear force. b) W_u – weight of the head and torso; L_u – lever arm of W_u about G (center of rotation of the knee); W_T – weight of the thigh; L_T – lever arm of W_T; W_A – weight of the arm; FQ – quadriceps force; $LQ = L_p = L_A$ – lever arms of FQ, P_A and W_A; JK – joint reaction force; CK – compression force; SK – shear force.

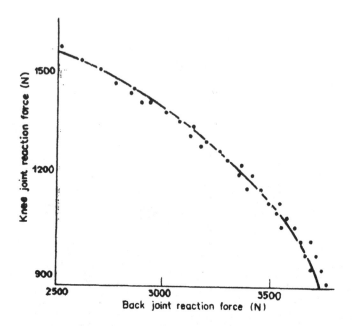

Fig. 3.20. Graph of the knee joint reaction force as a function of the
          back reaction force, when lifting position is allowed to vary.

a dynamic biomechanical model using actual segment motion data; to inves-

tigate the effect of box size on the weight of the load selected; to

validate the model by comparing predicted and measured ground reaction

forces and by correlating predicted low-back compressive forces external,

obtained from surface electromyography of the erector spinae muscles

measured during the lifts.

A seven links model (Fig. 3.21) is used. There are four steps in

resolving moments and forces on the body from the motion input data (i.e.

the X,Y, joint position data over time for the ankle, knee, hip, shoulder,

elbow and hand). The biomechanical data like masses, lengths of the links

based on average values taken from Drillis and Contini (1966) and Dempsten

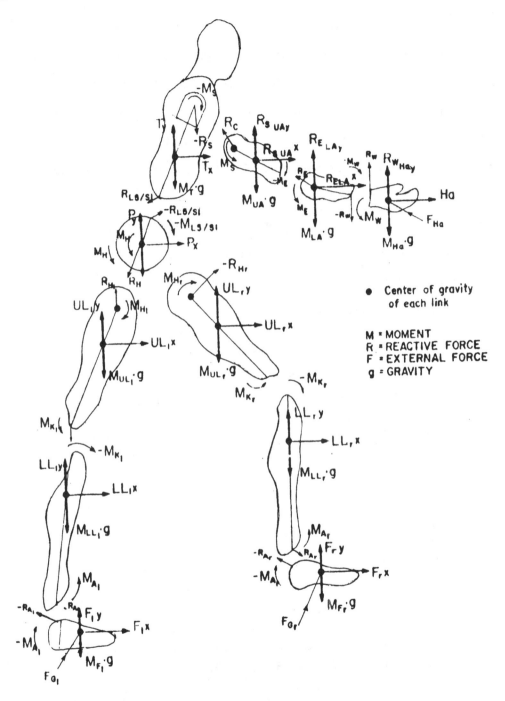

Fig. 3.21. Free body diagram of human body.

Six male subjects participated in the study. The subjects stood on a six-axis Kistler force platform which was connected on-line to an WP-2100 microcomputer. Monopolar surface electromyograph (EMa) recordings were obtained from the erector spinae muscles at the I_3/I_4 level. A plot of predicted ground reaction forces vs time into lift is shown in Fig. 3.22. A plot predicted L_5/S_1 compressive forces vs time into lift is shown in Fig. 3.23.. The basic conclusions are as follows:

- vertical ground reaction forces and predicted L_5/S_1 compressive in-
  creased with increasing load and with increasingly larger boxes;
- smoothed and rectified EMG correlated significantly with predicted
  L_5/S_1 compressive forces.

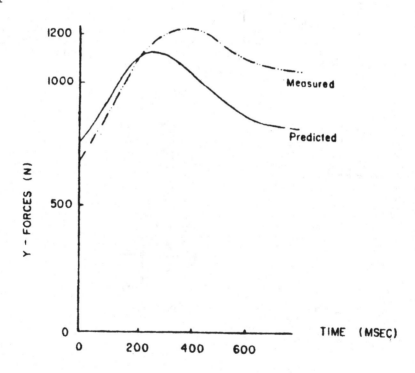

Fig. 3.22. Predicted and measured ground reaction forces (Y).

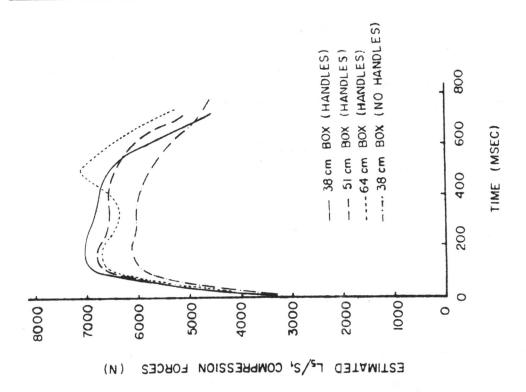

Fig. 3.23. Predicted L_5/S_1 compressive forces.

The last problem, which will be presented in this chapter will concern the calculation on mechanical power and mechanical efficiency during
distance running. Because widely verying estimates of mechanical power
have been calculated for a given speed of running by previous investigators, the effects of various assumptions necessary for mechanical power
calculations were evaluated via segmental energy analysis using 3D cine
data from 31 well trained subjects running overground at 3.37 ms^{-1} by
Williams and Cavanagh[20] in 1983.

Table 3.1 summizes the results of a number of studies which have
produced measures of mechanical power during running (speed ~3.57 ms^{-1}).

Table 3.1. A survey of mechanical power values obtained in previous studies calculated using a variety of computational methods. In
some cases the data were extracted from graphs and should only
be considered approximations. Original units have been con-
verted to watts.

	Method[*]	Approx. speed (ms^{-1})	Mechanical power (W)
Fukunaga et al. (1978)	1	3.6	343
Cavanga et al. (1977)	2	3.6	556
Norman et al. (1976)	3	3.6	172
Gregor & Kirkendall (1978)	3	3.6	163
Luhtanen & Komi (1978)	3	3.9	931
Luhtanen & Komi (1980)	3	3.9	1650
Winter (1979)	4	1.4	147
Pierrynowski et al. (1980)	4	1.5	166
Zarrugh (1981)	5	1.5	71

[*] The various methods used were: 1. Center of mass (c.m.) alone; 2. c.m.
+ movement of limbs relative to c.m.; 3. Pseudowork; 4. Segmental analysis; Walking.

It is obvious from table 3.1 that an extremely wide range for mechanical
power has been found previously for running at a approximately 3.6 ms^{-1},
even when using the same computational method for determining power. The
study which was carried on by Williams and Cavanagh examined the mechanical power generated in distance running at a speed of 3.57 ms^{-1} by
using a variety of computational methods. The effects of assumptions in-
volving the relative cost of positive and negative work, the contribu-
tions of energy transfer and the influence of elastic storage of energy
are considered. The basic segmetal methodology has been modified. Main
patterns of energy change from 31 subjects for individual segments are
shown in Fig.3.24 over the entire running cycle.

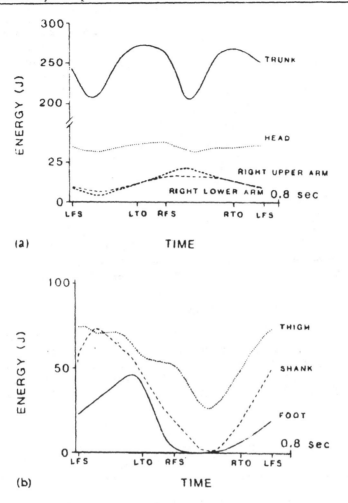

Fig. 3.24. Mean instantaneous segmental energy patterns from 31 subjects
during one complete running cycle for the a) head, trunk,
right upper arm, and forearm, and b) right thigh, shank and
foot.

Figure 3.25 shows mean instantaneous $NETPTR_i$ values during a half
cycle of running plotted against time for each of the four among segment
energy transfer criteria.

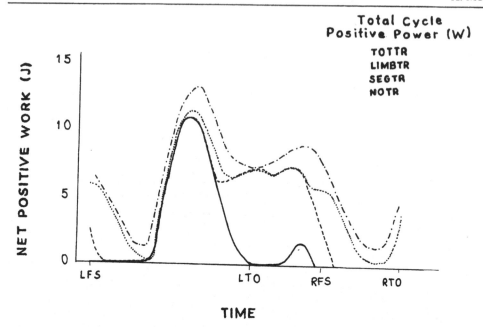

Fig. 3.25. Net positive work during the running cycle as determined
          using four different criteria for between segment energy
          transfer, ranging from complete transfer (TOTTR) to no
          transfer (NOTR). Positive power over the entire running
          cycle is also listed for each energy transfer method.

A method of determining mechanical power and efficiency (η) of running in the 1000 m was proposed by Ostrowska[21](1984) (Ph.D. dissertation
under Morecki's supervision). Eleven link model was used for calculation
of potential, kinematic and rotational energy of each segment of the model. The mechanical efficiency during running was calculated from the
formula

$$\eta = \frac{L_{u_b}}{L_{w_b}}$$
(3.11)

where L_{u_b} is internal work produced by runner during running; L_{w_b} is input
work (energetical cost of running) calculated from oxygen consumption dur-

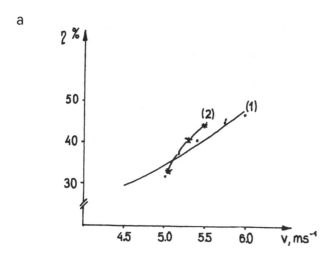

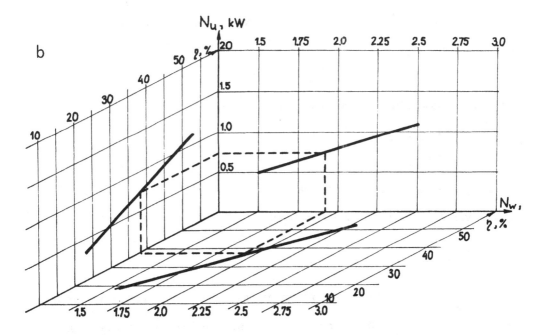

Fig. 3.26. Main results obtained during running the distance 1000 m.
a – mechanical efficency as a function of velocity of running
b – nomogram N_w, N_u η for distance 1000 m.

ing the activity and 20 minutes rest.

Computer analysis of cinematohraphic technic of registration was used. The films were analyzed with a NAC photoanalyzer and digitized by PDP 11/34 computer. Six man subjects aged 21–24 were tested three times during the 1000 m runs with constant speed between 5–6 ms^{-1}. Figure 3.26a presents the relationship between efficiency η and the velocity of running (v). In the frame of velocity between 5–6 ms^{-1} the best approximation was obtained from formula

$$\eta = \sqrt{318.7v^2 - 2388.8v + 5166} \qquad (3.12)$$

The coefficient of correlation was r = 0.677 on level $\alpha < 0.01$. The relationship between useful power, input power and efficiency η is presented in Fig. 3.26b. It is enough to know one parameter only for calculation the two others.

MANIPULATION AND LOCOMOTION PROBLEMS

This chapter contains the following problems:

- animal locomotion;

- walking machines;

- control aspects of artificial hands;

- upper and lower extremity FMS and FNS.

Animal locomotion and walking machines

The whole of an animal's locomotory machinery can, like that of a motor car, be divided into three main parts, namely: the engine, the transmission gear and the propeller (Gray[22]). The muscles constitute the engine or prime mover converting internal chemical energy into mechanical energy. The transmission elements of a vertebrate animal are the bones operating as levers; the propeller is that part of the animal's surface which exerts its effort against the external environment.

The animal can adjust the length and height of its steps to meet irregularities of the ground and to break the shock of impact with the ground. The limb is equivalent to a wheel whose diameter can be varried and where the vehicle is fitted with very powerful shock absorber.

The feasibility of applying the principle of jointed limbs for the propulsion of land vehicles over rough country has been discussed by Shigley (1961), who concluded that each wheel of a self-propelled vehicle can be replaced by four "feet" placed on the ground in sequence with one--quarter of a cycle difference in phase between each "foot"; to replace four wheels, four groups each with four feet would be required, and the timing of a hind group would have to be coordinated with that of a front group (Fig. 4.1). The energy required for vertebrate locomotion is devided from striated muscle fibres. The output of mechanical power depends of the rate (v) of which a fibre shortens against a given load (P). The conditions under which a muscle yields a maximum amount of mechanical po-

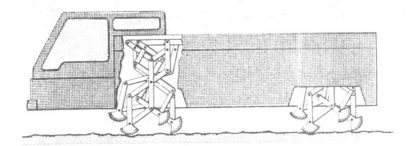

Fig. 4.1. Drawing of a panto-graph-legged vehicle using hydraulic power.

wer have been clearly defined by Hill (1950). Those problems were devel-

oped next by Wilkie[23] (1960).

The body of a terrestrial tetrapod can be regarded as a loaded flex-

ible beam supported and propelled by four extensible limbs range of move-

ment and posture is largely determined by the over-riding affect of the

weight of the body (Gray, 1944). According to Gray, from an evolutionary

point of view, it would be logical to start with the limbs of amphibians

and trace the changes which occured first in reptiles and then in mammals.

From a mechanical point of ciew, however, the body and limbs of a typical

cursorial mammal are in two respects considerably simpler than those of

amphibia or reptiles. The constituant joints and bones of the limb all

lie in or near a single vertical longitudinal plane passing through the

shoulder or hip joint. When the animal is in motion the movement of the

limb relative to the body is also restricted to this plane. As illustrated

in Fig. 4.2 and Fig. 4.3, the body of animal such as a horse can be com-

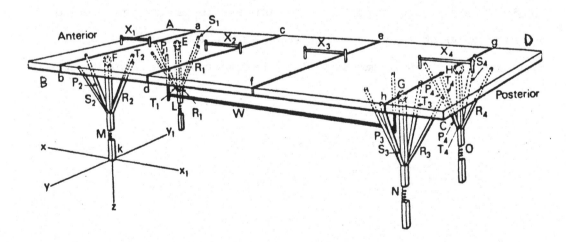

Fig. 4.2. Diagram of a table illustrating the general relationship between the muscles and skeleton of a tetrapod.

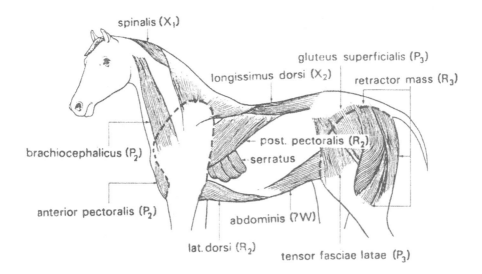

spinalis (X_1)

gluteus superficialis (P_3)

longissimus dorsi (X_2)

retractor mass (R_3)

brachiocephalicus (P_2)

post. pectoralis (R_2)

serratus

anterior pectoralis (P_2)

abdominis (?W)

lat. dorsi (R_2)

tensor fasciae latae (P_3)

Fig. 4.3. Diagram showing the functional relationship of some of the
extrinsic limb muscles and axial muscles of the horse to the
braces shown in figure 4.2.

pared with a table whose constituant part are hinged to their neigbours

and held in position by elastic braces. The detailed description of the

ability of limbs to exert vertical forces against the body, equilibrium

of external forces acting on the body, limbs operated as levers, stability

relationship of muscular effort to external environment can be found in

some works[22,23].

An interesting description on different aspects of animal mechanics

is given by McNeil Alexander[23] and Raibert and Sutherland[24]. Based on

some geometrical, kinematical and dynamical properties of insects and

vertebrate motion, many different walking machines were designed. Four

of most fascinating projects running at present are shown in Fig. 4.4 a,

b, c and d, namely, the advanced hopping machine developed by Raibert

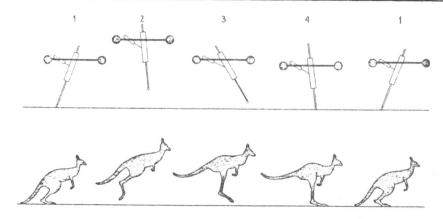

Fig. 4.4a. Hopper in motion.

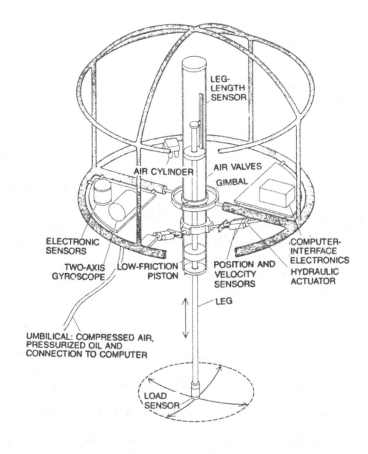

Fig. 4.4b. Advanced hopping machine.

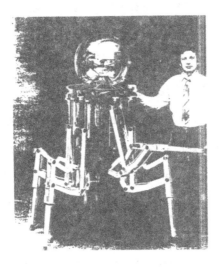

c)

Figure 1.7.9.1.(5) Odex I vehicle (Odetics,USA,1983): 1,leg created from a parallelogram 1 to 2 and 3 to 4, with strict class 1 structure;5, rod for control of upper leg(3 to 4). The control rod for the lower leg is is hidden further inside the vehicle;

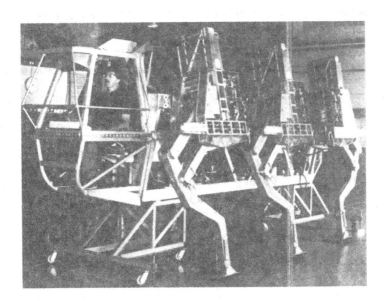

d)

Fig.4.4 ASV 85(Adaptive suspension vehicle)

Carnagie-Melon University, USA, 1983, (Fig. 4.4 a and b), Odex I vehicle
(Odetics, USA, 1983) (Fig. 4.4c) and ASV 84 (Adaptive Suspension Vehicle
by Ohio State University, USA, 1985) (Fig. 4.4d).[25,26]

A programme concerning the design of four legged walking machines
started a few years ago at the Team of Biomechanics, Technical University
of Warsaw (Jaworek, Pogorzelski, Zielinska). Some latest results obtained
by Zielinska (1985) - part of her Ph.D. dissertation will be presented.
Three computer programmes concerning different kinds of walk was elabo-
rated[27].

The first programme "par" is concern with the calculation of parameters of the walk during the movements on slope, the second one "slop"
to visualize the walk of the machine on the slope, and the third one for
calculation and visualization of so-called balancing stages of machine.

We will briefly discuss the problem of balancing. We assume that the
machine is in a such situation that the position of its legs are not in
according with the gait programme. We will determine the movements which
must be realize by the machine to achive the previous position, without
loosing the stability. The initial state, in a wrong position, is a four
legged state. The final state according to the gait programme, will be
three legged state. It is necessary during the balancing process (Fig.4.5)
to realize four movements, namely:

- change of the leg position (state 1),

- displacement of the body of the machine (state 2),

- change of the other leg (state 3),

- displacement of the body of machine (state 4).

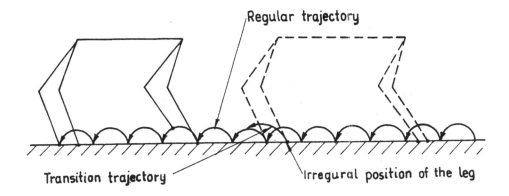

Regular trajectory

Transition trajectory

Irregural position of the leg

Fig. 4.5. Balancing process of four legged machine.

CONTROL ASPECTS OF ARTIFICIAL HANDS AND UPPER AND LOWER EXTREMITIES

FUNCTIONAL NEUROMUSCULAR STIMULATION

According to the statistical data, about 10 to 12% of population in the developed countries are disabled people and half of them needs an assistance of special devices for substituting or supporting the lost functions in manipulation and locomotion activity. In the last years, independently from prosthetics-orthotics direction new trends in the design and application of different types of manipulators, which anable the patients to contact the world while being at home and permit him to carry out some working activity, can be observed.

The rehabilitation manipulator we shall define as a bionic mechanism partially anthropomorphic, designed to perform – in a stated range – the functions of man's upper extremity (Fig. 5.1a). The mani-pedipulative system we shall define as an assembly of bionic mechanisms, partially anthropomorphic, designed to perform – in a stated range – the functions of both upper and lower extremities associated with patient's service (Fig. 5.1b) (Morecki, 1984). But that also be of the type directly.

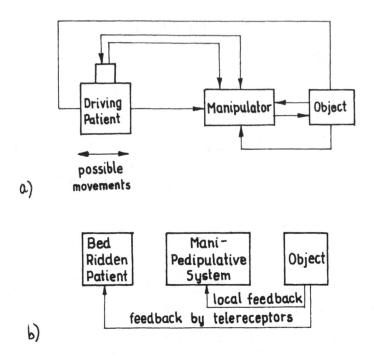

Fig. 5.1. Rehabilitiation systems. a – rehabilitation manipulator;
          b – mani–pedipulative system.

connected to the patient, though not to the stump. At the Design Division

of Stanford University and the Palo Alto Veterans Administration Hospital

spinal cord injury service a rehabilitation system[28] using SMART robotic

arms with multi-processor control system was designed. The structure of

this system is shown in Fig. 5.2. A rehabilitation manipulator designed

by J.Ober directly connected to the patient (mounted on the head) is shown

in Fig. 5.3.[26,28] The description of many other solutions of rehabilita-

tion manipulators are given in many books[25,26].

But still the key question of the future development is not clear

specially from the·point of view of the patient. Another interesting meth-

od for supporting of the lost functions both in manipulation and locomo-

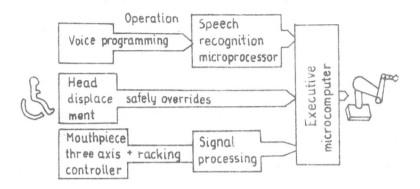

Fig. 5.2. Structure of the system.

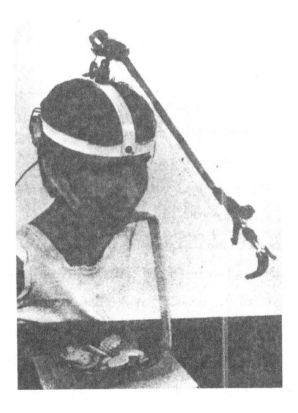

Fig. 5.3. Head manipulator.

tion activity is so-called Functional Neuromuscular Stimulation specially

using in cases of spinal cord injury. This method provides a mechanism

for the activation of muscles paralyzed by injury to the spinal cord.This

technique was first used over 20 years ago. Only recent advances in ele-

ctronics and biomechanics have made it a promissing aid for rehabilitation

of these patients. Restoration of grasping movements, standing and biped

gait in paraplegics has been achieved under carefully controlled laborato-

ry conditions[29,.30,31,32,33].

SELECTED PROBLEMS

Four selected problems of modern biomechanics will be presented,

namely:

- man under vibration,

- model of dynamic cooperation of muscles,

- design of anthropomorphic manipulators,

- design and application of "alive" manipulators.

In the first area we will discuss two problems:

- the mechanical behaviour of active human skeletal muscle in small oscil-

lations (Cannon, Zahalak; 1982)[34];

- man under vibration mathematical model and analysis (Nader, 1984)[35].

The experimental results concerning the small amplitude dynamic response

of muscle in vivo will be discussed. The proposed model represents the

perturbation response of the forearm flexion-extension system about a sta-

te of steady isometric contraction. The model is quasi-linear, having the

form of a linear differential equation. For a single muscle the model has

the structure shown in Fig. 6.1, and represents the muscle as a two input

(length perturbation and activation - EMG perturbation) one output (force

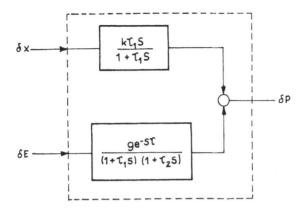

$$\delta x \longrightarrow \boxed{\dfrac{k\tau_1 S}{1+\tau_1 S}}$$

$$\longrightarrow \delta P$$

$$\delta E \longrightarrow \boxed{\dfrac{g e^{-s\tau}}{(1+\tau_1 s)(1+\tau_2 s)}}$$

Fig. 6.1. Block diagram of muscle model.

perturbation) system. This model may be used to predict the system re-

sponse measured in frequency-response experiments. A schematic diagram

of the experiment used in this investigation is shown in Fig. 6.2. Five

static tests were applied to each subject. As a result of the analysis

all seven model parameters have been identified and the forced oscilla-

tion test's (FOT's) response was re-examined to check the accuracy of the

model perdictions. This is illustrated in Fig. 6.3 where the perdictions

of equation are compared with the measured frequency response.

Mathematical models of the standing and a seating man under vibra-

tion was analysed by Nader[35] (1984) as a part of his Ph.D. dissertation.

Two above mentioned models are shown in Figs 6.4 and 6.5. In the first

case $Z_1 \div Z_{12}$ are the vertical mass center of displacement of the parts of

the body and Z_p is vertical displacement of the floor, k_i and C_i are

stiffness and dumping consecutivly. In the second case (Fig. 6.5) $Z_1 \div Z_9$

are the vertical displacements of the part of the body and Z_s is vertical

displacement of the seat. The equations of motion for the bio-dynamical

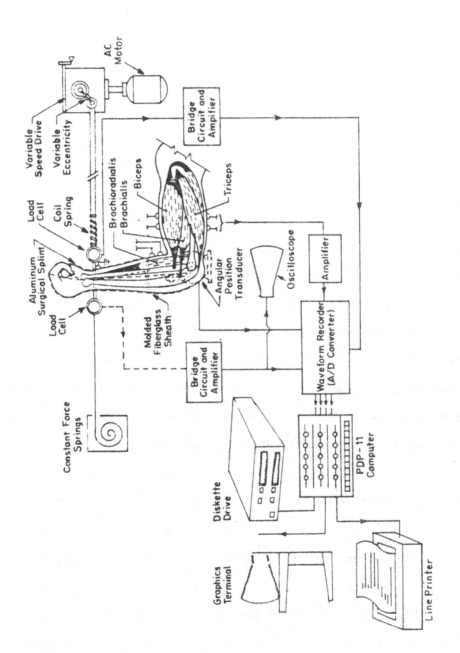

Fig. 6.2. Schematic diagram of experimental arrangement.

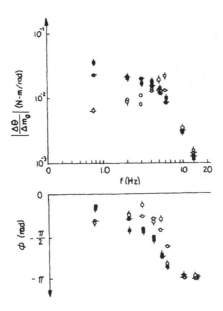

Fig. 6.3. Comparison of observed FOT frequency response to that predicted muscle model, using measured EMG. For the sake of clarity, only the highest and lowest mean contraction levels are shown; fitted squares = 74 Nm, open circles = 26 Nm. Horizontal marks indicate measured data points. Vertical marks indicate the model response using the measured feedback EMG as an input. Each point is the mean of two repetitions at the given frequency.

models have been desired by the method of forces.

The dynamical behaviour of the mathematical model was investigated by computing of

- the eigen values and vectors,

- the transmittance matrix,

- the dynamic transfer function,

- the parametric sensitiveness of eigen values.

A series of tests have been proceeded for assesing the vertical vibration components in the driver's cabin of an electric locomotive (EN-57, widely

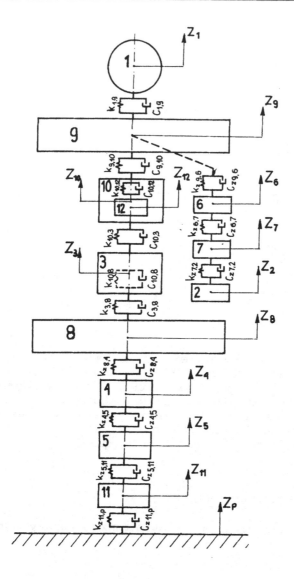

Fig. 6.4. Standing man under vibration model.

used in Poland for suburban shuttle train service).

The example of vibration spectrum is shown in Fig. 6.6 together with respective acceleration limits the ISO 2631 – 1978 (E) Standard.

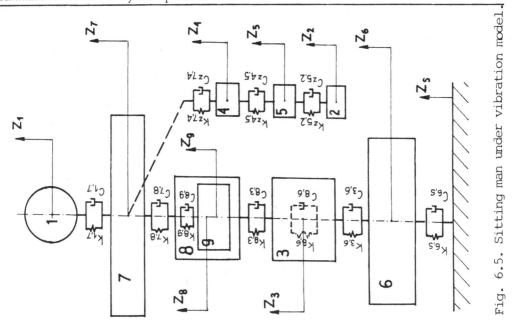

Fig. 6.5. Sitting man under vibration model.

Fig. 6.3. Comparison of observed FOT frequency response to that predicted
by the muscle model, using measured EMG. (These data are for

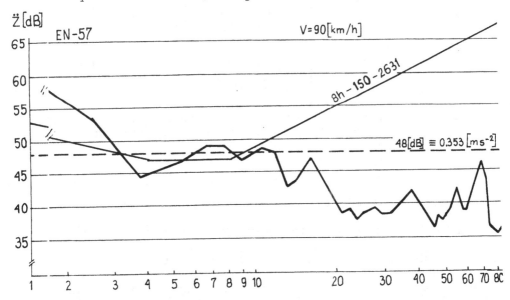

Fig. 6.6. RMS acceleration of cabin floor vs frequency. AT V=90 km/h
the vehicle fails to meet the ISO-2631 8-hour criterion at
3.1 Hz and over the frequency band 5.4 to 8.2 Hz.

Item	Organs or structures		Frequency basis where vibration is amplified maximum gain and peak frequency (theoretical) (Hz)	Spot frequencies and frequency bands of recorded vehicle vibration (Hz)	Spot frequencies and frequency bands where man noxiously cited to vibration (Hz)
	Input	Output			
1	buttox	int.abdomen organs	1.2 to 5.4 max. gain 3.1x at 3.0 Hz	2.6	2.6
2	upper torso	head	12.0 to 41.0 max. gain 2.8x at 34.0 Hz	6–8	14–16
3	upper torso	hands	1.5 to 17.0 max. gain 2.7x at 11.0 Hz	10–11	2.6, 6–8, 10–11, 14–
4	upper torso	forearms	1.4 to 16.0 max. gain 2.7x at 11.0 Hz	14–16	2.6, 6–8, 10–11, 14–
5	buttox	chest	1.0 to 8.9 max. gain 2.2x at 5.2 Hz	46–51	2.6, 6–
6	buttox	int. chest organs	1.0 to 15.5 max. gain 2.0 at 5.0 Hz	64–68	2.6, 6–, 10–11, 14–

Table 6.1.   Underlined spot frequencies and frequency bands are those deemed of most importance for the vibration of analyzed organs or structures of man.

Table 6.1 shows an example (seating man) of comparison between theoretical most noxious frequency bands with those spot frequencies and frequency bands where highest accelerations were recorded at the cabin floor. Most affected are the driver's head, the abdominal organs, internal chest organs and upper limbs and the driver's exposure exceeds the "decreased proficiency boundary".

The next problem to be discussed is concern the model of dynamic co-operation of muscles operated the elbow joint in the fast flexion and extension movements. The model of muscle cooperation in dynamical conditions was presented in some papers[36, 37]. The joint was treated as an element of automatic control system with linear part located in the main loop and with non-linear part in the feedback loop. An example of cooperation of the muscles operated elbow joint during flexion was solved. A good correlation between the external moment and the sum of torques of individual muscles was obtained.

We will shortly discuss elbow joint as a joint with one degree of freedom only, operated by a set of seven muscles actons, namely four flexors (BBCL, B, BBCB, BR) and three extensors (TBCL, TBCLat and TBCM). The mathematical model negligible the damping, can be presented in the given below form (Fig. 6.7)

$$ J\ddot{\alpha} - (\sum_1^4 M_{fi} - \sum_1^3 M_{exi}) = 0 , \qquad (6.1)$$

where J is mass moment of inertia of the forearm and hand according to the axis of the joint, perpendicular to the plane of motion (constant dur-

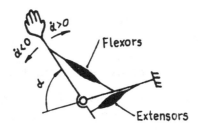

Fig. 6.7 Mathematical model of the muscles operated elbow joint

ing the motion); $\ddot{\alpha}$ is angular acceleration; M_{fi} and M_{exi} are the muscle
torque exerted concecutively by the flexors and extensors.

The equation (6.1) holds for the range of the joint angle $\alpha_{min} < \alpha < \alpha_{max}$
The first formulation of the problem of muscle cooperation in quasi-dyna-
mic movement was given by A.Morecki and others[36]. Next the investigations
of muscle cooperation operating the angle joint in flexion were carried
out by K.Kedzior[36]. Based on those results the next step in the area of
mathematical modelling of muscle cooperation in fast movements was done
by E.Bieżanowska[37]. In Dabrowska's work[38] new results are obtained concern
ing the relationship between force and integrated EMG based on dynamical
model. In this paper some of the latest results will be discussed. The
torque M in equation (6.1) can be described in a form

$$M = u \cdot f_s(\alpha) \cdot f_d(\dot{\alpha}) \; f_i(t) \; r(\alpha) \qquad\qquad (6.2)$$

where u is variable excitation from 0 to 1; $f_s(\alpha)$ is force-angle relation
under static conditions for maximum excitation; $f_d(\dot{\alpha})$ is relationship between force developed in dynamical conditions and velocity or rotatory
motion of the joint; $f_i(t)$ are delay functions of muscle force response
to excitation; $r(\alpha)$ is moment arm developed on the angle of rotation in
a joint. If we assume $\alpha = x_1$ and $\dot{\alpha} = x_2$ from equations (6.1) and (6.2) we
obtain

$$\underline{x} = f(x, u, t) , \qquad\qquad (6.3)$$

where $\underline{x}$ is state vector; $\underline{u}$ is control vector and t is time. Assuming that
at the beginning of motion, for $t_p = 0$ the value of state vector $\underline{x}_p = \begin{vmatrix} x_{1p} \\ x_{2p} \end{vmatrix}$
and at the end $t = t_k$, $\underline{x}_k = \begin{vmatrix} x_{1k} \\ x_{2k} \end{vmatrix}$ the motion in a joint can be determined

as a change of the vector $\underline{x}$ from $\underline{x}_p$ to $\underline{x}_k$ in the frame $t_p \leqslant t \leqslant t_k$.

If we are interested in the fast movements, it means the movements performed in a minimum of time, the following conditions should be fulfilled

$$t_k - t_p = \min. \tag{6.4}$$

The solution of this problem needs to find such an excitation values of muscles that is state vector $\underline{u}$, that the solution of equation (6.3) by conditions $\underline{x}_p$ and $\underline{x}_k$ fulfill the requirements (6.4). We obtain a typical optimal problem to be solved.

The solution of minimum-time motion problem, that is the determining of the state vector $\underline{u}$ can be performed through calculation of the optimal value of the quality index V. From the Bellman condition

$$- \frac{\partial V}{\partial t} = \min_{\underline{u}} H. \tag{6.5}$$

On the basis of analysis (Jacobsen, 1970; Findeisen, 1974) the linearity of the Hamiltonian with respect to the control set $\underline{u}$ was assumed, and therefore the optimal control for the motion can assume boundary values either 0 or 1. So, the problem of dynamic programming is reduced to the problem of optimization in statics (Gawronski, 1980). The quality index of the control expressed as

$$V = w(\max t_{ij} + t_d) + \sum_1^2 w_i (x_{fi} - x_i | \underline{u}, t_f (\underline{u}) |)^2 \tag{6.6}$$

where $\max t_{ij}$ is maximum total time for all switching of the i-th muscle; t_d is time of stopping the motion ($\&=0$), after all the control signals are switched off; w, w_i are dimensional weights converting the quality index to the dimensionless form; x_{fi} are required terminal values of the state

vector, this is the angle of rotation in a joint and the velocity;

$x_i|\underline{u},t_f(\underline{u})|$ are values of the state vactor for the final time t_f (if

$t_f(\underline{u}) = t_f(u_{opt}) = t_{f\,min}$ then $x_i|\underline{u},t_f(\underline{u})| = x_{fi}$); r is coefficient ful-

filling the condition (Findeisen, 1974), $\lim\limits_{r \to \infty} \min V = \min\limits_{\underline{u}} |(\max t_{ij}+t_d)\cdot w|$.

The expression $w(\max t_{ij}+t_d)$ is the basic quality index for the motion,

which has to be performed in a minimum time. The cost function is increa-

sed by the penalty function, which corresponds to limitations imposed on

the motion.

The experiment were performed on a test group of 8 young male subjects

and proved the repeatability of the charakter of the parameters $\alpha,\dot\alpha$, EMG

for fast flexion and extension. Then a computer simulation was performed

on a model, corresponding to one of the subjects. An own computer programme

JACOBS was used for calculations, which utilizes optimization procedure

MINUIT (James, Roos, 1977) based on the Nedler and Mead's and Davidson's

method. The equations of the process were solved by RKINIT procedure

(Runge-Kutta fourth-order) method. Due to a large number of optimized

parameters (24 switching times for 7 muscles) the computation time re-

quired for the assumed accuracy (resulting from the experiments) was

about 3 system hours for the CDC 6600 computer. The comparison of the real.

and the computed trajectories does not lead to rejection of the minimum

time criterion, followed by the living organism while performing quick

motions. Thus, the description of cooperation of muscles yieled by the

simulation can be accepted. Figure 6.8 shows an example of the comparison

mode for a quick extension of the extremity from 90° to 10°. The mean

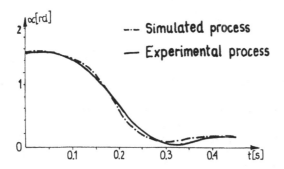

Fig. 6.8. Quick extension of the extremity from 90° to 10°. Comparison between experimental and the computed trajectories.

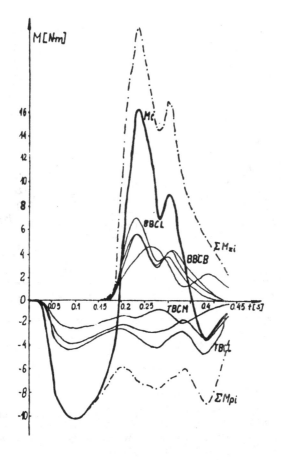

Fig. 6.9. Cooperation of seven muscles operated an elbow joint.

discrepencies between the experimental and the computed trajectories are less than the measured error for the angle (2°). The difference in time for real and computed trajectories is less than 6%.

Figure 6.9 shows the picture of cooperation of seven muscles and its comparison with total torque M_c, during the fast extension. The further development of the problem of cooperation of muscles in dynamical conditions was given by Zmyslowski[40] in 1980.

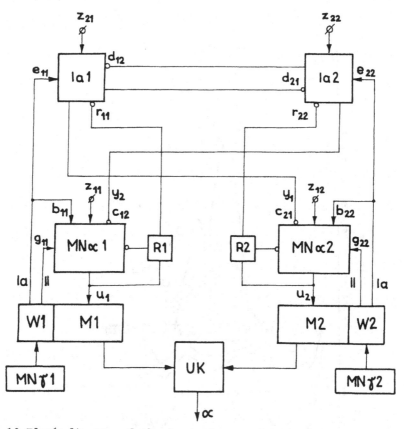

Fig.6.10 Block diagram of the basic loops of spinal level and neuronal elements connected with the pair of antagonistic muscles
$MN\alpha$ –motoneurons α, $M\gamma$ –motoneurons γ, W –receptors, R – Renshaw cells, I_a – interneurons Ia, M – muscle, U_k – skeleton system
$MN\alpha$ and $M\gamma$ are the activated feedback,W,R–blocking feedback

The dynamical model of the pair of antagonistic muscles operated the elbow joint was connected with the elements of motoneurons located in the feedback loops on spinal level (Fig. 6.10). The mathematical model was formulated. It consists of a set of non-linear equations, which describe the whole system. The influence of the feedback loops on the solution of a set of equations, which describe the state of the system close to equilibrium was investigated.

Design and control of anthropomorphic manipulators

The concept of anthropomorphism is defined here as a structural simi-larity of upper extremities of the man and the manipulator, as well as the correspondence of their basic dimensions. Moreover, it is assumed that the power output measured at particular joints is of the same order of the power output of a man performing typical manual work.

The structure and the drive system of the manipulator described by Morecki and Kedzior[39] is based on an open kinematic chain with six degrees of freedom (Fig. 6.11a). This manipulator is operated by a special system of electronically controlled mechanical amplifiers and incorporated dif-ferential gear with two degrees of freedom. The control system allows us to determine the relationship between the vector of forces exerted by the cables and the vector of control signals (Fig. 6.11b). The tension in the cable is controlled by means of an electromagnetic brake.

The investigations carried out in the last period of time were con-centrated on:

- mathematical description of an open kinematic chain with a few degrees of freedom;

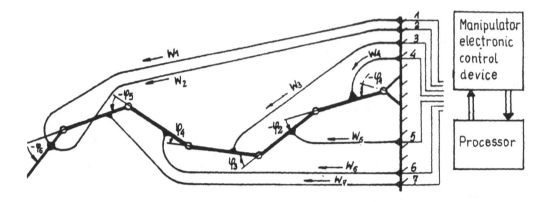

Fig.6.11. Model of anthropomorphic manipulator with six degrees
of freedom, w_1-w_7 - cables, φ_1 - φ_6 - service angles

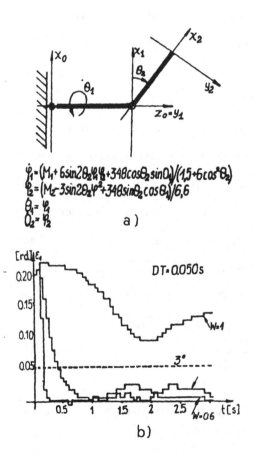

a)

b)

Fig.6.12 Model of manipula
tor with two degr
ees of freedom(a)
max.deviation
from a given traj
ectory (b)

- realization of control algorithms for performing a given trajectory;

- digital simulation of a mechanical system with a few degrees of freedom
  with a goal to determine the maximum deviations from the given trajectory, which allows the returning to present trajectory, (Fig. 6.12).
  Figure 6.12a shows the mechanical model of two degrees of freedom manipulator for digital simulation and equations of motion, and Fig. 6.12b
  shows process of control for different weights w; stable for w=0.6,
  unstable for w=1;

- designing of the new, more efficient drive unit specially for a control
  of multijoint cable actuators;

- design of a microprocessor system of control for this kind of manipulators.

Design and application of "alive" manipulators

The results obtained in the years 1971-1985 with the use of implanted
stimulators of nerves for forcing grasping activities of paralyzed upper
extremities of arm looks very promising for rehabilitation engineering.

The medium nerve (medianus) was stimulated with use of implanted
stimulators in order to obtain a grasping function of the hand. In several
cases, the radial nerve (radialis) was also stimulated with a view to
increase hand opening. In the years 1976-81 a new conception of the hybrid
system of forcing of the grasping movements was designed and tested under
clinical conditions.

This system was realized under condition of simultaneous cooperation
of a patient with the system of stimulators implanted on the nerves combined with the external orthosis. Figure 6.13a shows the sequence of the

activities in the grasping movement and an example of technical solution.

Tests were carried on four patients with spinal cord injury of C6 level

by implanting two stimulators on the median and radial nerves.

Orthosis with the position transducer installed in the metacarpo-

phelanged joint was mounted on the right extremity. The obtained records

of the changes in the angle of the palm opening and closing as a function

of time show that the motion is mild and relatively smooth (Fig. 6.13b,c).

It is hoped that the hybrid system proposed for supporting of the lost

grasping movements enables the patient to provide the every day activity

and accelerates the rehabilitation process. Based on these promising re-

sults a new project was started in 1982. It is combining in one multi-

functional apparatus the possibilities of simultaneous nerves, pain and

bones stimulation. It is expected by using such a device to accelerate

bone growth after damage with parallel decrease of pain influence[39].

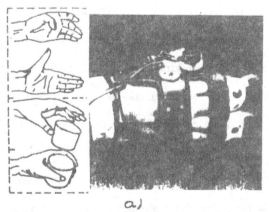

a)

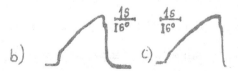

b)   c)

Fig. 6.13. "Alive" manipulator. a) the sequence of movements; b) obtained
results.

REFERENCES

1. Morecki, A., Ekiel, J. and Fidelus, K., *Cybernetic systems of limb movements in man, animals and robots*, PWN-Polish Scientific Publishers Warsaw and Ellis Horwood Limited Publishers, Chichester, 1984, 8.

2. Baildon, R.W.A. and Chapman, E.A., A new approach to the human muscle model, *J. of Biomechanics*, 16, 10, 803, 1983.

3. Petrofsky, J.S. and Phillips, C.A., The influence of temperature, initial length and electrical activity of the force-velocity relationship of the medical gastrocnemius muscle of the cat, *J. of Biomechanics*, 14, 5, 297, 1981.

4. Lago, P.J. and Jones, N.B., Parameter estimation of system dynamics with modulation-type noise - application to the modelling of the dynamic relationship between the EMG and force transients in muscle, in *IEE Proc.*, 131, P.D., 6, 1984, 221.

5. Polit, A. and Bizzi, E., Process controlling arm movements in monkeys, in *Science*, Am. Assoc. for the Advancement of Science, Washington, 1978, 1235.

6. Gandy, M. et al., Acquisition and analysis of electromyographic data associated with dynamic movements of the arm, *Medical and Biological Engineernig and Computing*, 57, 1980.

7. Morosso, P., Spatial control of arm movements, in *Experimental brain research*, Springer Verlag, 1981, 223.

8. Fried, I. et al., Organization of visurspatial functions in human cortex, evidence from electrical stimulation, *Brain*, 349, 1982.

9. Hammond, G.R., Miller, S. and Robertson, P.M., Central nervous control of arm movements in stroke patients, in *Brain stem control of spinal*

mechanisms, Elsevier Biomedical Press, 1982, 324.

10. Morawski, J.M., Model studies of the pole vault, Report 1977, MINS, AWF, Warsaw, 1977 (in Polish).

11. Hubbard, M., Dynamics of the pole vault, *J. of Biomechanics*, 13, 11, 965, 1980.

12. Morawski, J., Article in *J. of Biomechanics*, 6, 1975.

13. Remizov, L.P., Optimal running on skis in downhill, *J.of Biomechanics* 13, 11, 941, 1980.

14. Maryniak J., Static and dynamic investigations of human motion, in *Mechanics of Biological Solids, Euromech. Colloquium 68*, Bulgarian Academy of Sciences, Sofia, 1977.

15. Remizov, L.P., Biomechanics of optimal flight in ski-jumping, *J. of Biomechanics*, 17, 3, 167, 1984.

16. Dapena, J., Simulation of modified human airborne movements, *J. of Biomechanics*, 14, 2, 81, 1981.

17. Gervalis, P. and Marino, G.M., A procedure for determining angular positional data relative to the principal axes of the human body, *J. of Biomechanics*, 16, 2, 109, 1983.

18. Bejjani, F.J., Gross, C.M. and Pugh, J.W., Model for static lifting: relationship of loads on the spine and the knee, *J. of Biomechanics*, 17, 4, 284, 1984.

19. Freivalds, A. et al., A dynamic biomechanical evaluation of lifting maximum acceptable loads, *J. of Biomechanics*, 17, 4, 251, 1984.

20. Williams, K.R. and Cavanagh, P.R., A model for the calculation of biomechanical power during distance running, *J. of Biomechanics*, 16, 2, 115, 1983.

21. Ostrowska, E., The method of calculation of mechanical efficiency of runners in 1000 m running, Ph.D. dissertation, Academy of Physical Education, Warsaw, 1984.

22. Gray, J., *Animal Locomotion*, Weidenfeld and Nicolson, London W1.

23. McNeil Alexander, R., *Animal Mechanics*, Blockwell Scientific Publications, Oxford-London

24. Raibert, M.H. and Sutherland, I.E., Machines that walk, *Scientific American*, 248, 44, 1983.

25. Vertut, J. and Coiffet, P., Robot technology, in *Teleoperation and Robotics, Evolution and Development*, Hermes Publishing, Paris, 1984.

26. *Proc. of Ro.man.sy' 84, The Fifth CISM-IFToMM Symposium on Theory and Practice of Robots and Manipulators*, Morecki, A., Bianchi, G. and Kedzior, K. (Eds.), Kogan Page, London, Hermes Publishing, Paris,1985.

27. Zielinska, T., Synthesis and control of four legged machine, Ph.D. dissertation, Warsaw University of Technology (in preparation).

28. Morecki, A., Control Aspects of Artificial Hand, in *Control Aspects of Biomedical Engineering, Trends and Progress*, IFAC Monographs (in printing).

29. Weiss, M. et al., An electronical hybrid device for the control of hand functions by electrical stimulation methods, in *Biomechanics* VII-A University Park Press, Baltimore, Polish Scientific Publishers, Warsaw, 1981, 397.

30. Morecki, A. et al., A new method for forcing lost grasping functions ted of extremities by use of an orthotic manipulator combined with implanted stimulators of nerves, in *Proc. of Int. Conf. on Medical Devices and Sport Equipment*, August 18-21, 1980, San Francisco, USA.

31. Morecki, A., Methodology and technical aids for substituting of upper human extremities - where are we going?, in *Biomechanics VIII-A*,Human Kinetic Publishers, Champaign, 1983, 341.

32. Morecki, A. and Borowski, H., On one system applied to support the lost functions of prehension movement, in *Proc. of the 1st Vienna Int. Workshop on Functional Electrostimulation*, Vienna, Oct.19-21, 1983.

33. Cybulski, C.R., Penu, R.D. and Jaeger, R.J., Lower extremity functional neuromuscular stimulation in cases of spinal cord injury, *Neurosurgery*, 15, 1, 1984.

34. Cannon, S.C. and Zaholak, G.I., The mechanical behaviour of active human skeletal muscle in small oscillations, *J. of Biomechanics*, 15, 2, 111, 1982.

35. Bajon, W. and Nader, M., The analysis of locomotive drivers reaction on certain dynamical loads, in *Proc. 2nd Int. CISM-IFToMM Symp. "Man under Vibration"*, Moscow, April 8-12,1985, 139.

36. *Biomechanics of Motion, CISM Cources and Lectures No. 263*, Morecki A. (Ed.), Springer Verlag, Wien, New York, 1980.

37. Bieżanowska, E., Modelling of muscle cooperation under dynamical conditions (in Polish), Ph.D. dissertation, Warsaw University of Technology, 1982.

38. Morecki, A. et al., Cooperation of muscles under dynamic conditions with stimulation control, in *Control Aspects of Prosthetics and Orthotics /IFAC Symp./*, Pergamon Press, 1983, 7.

39. Morecki, A. and Kedzior, K., Dynamic modelling and synthesis of biomechanical system, in *Proc. of SCSC´84*, July 23-25, 1984, Boston, Vol. 2, 840.

40. Zmysłowski, W., Selected problems of muscle control synthesis; information processing on spinal cord level, Institute for Cybernetics and Biomedical Engng., Polish Academy of Sciences, Preprint, 18, 1984.

CALCULATION OF LOADS TRANSMITTED AT THE ANATOMICAL JOINTS

N. Berme, G. Heydinger and A. Cappozzo*
The Ohio State University, Columbus, Ohio, U.S.A.
*Università degli Studi "La Sapienza", Roma, Italy

INTERSEGMENTAL LOADS

At present there exists no practical method to directly measure the loads acting on the structures associated with in-vivo anatomical joints. These loads must be estimated from a knowledge of the resultant intersegmental loading at the joint. With the resultant loading at the joint known, a mathematical model of the joint system can be devised in an attempt to predict the loads acting on the associated muscles, ligaments, and joint surfaces.

Intersegmental forces and couples can be calculated, using measurable quantities and analytical mechanics. This is achieved through the following sequence of operations:

a) development of a mechanical model of the relevant parts of the human body,

b) selection of the model parameters (inertia properties)

c) selection of a set of quantities (variables) that completely describe the mechanical behavior of the model and that are

measurable on a living subject while the physical exercise under
investigation is being executed (kinematic and external loading
quantities)

d) identification of the mathematical equations which permit the
    calculation of the intersegmental actions using the model
    parameters and measured quantities as input variables (solution
    of the inverse dynamics problem)

e) experimental assessment of these quantities and parameters, and

f) calculation of the intersegmental forces and couples.

This approach requires the use of simplifying assumptions about the
mechanical structure and behavior of the human body. Thus, the accuracy
of the intersegmental force and couple calculations is limited not only
by the quality of the input data, but also by the validity of these
simplifying assumptions. Without a fairly accurate knowledge of the
intersegmental loads, further modeling and calculations in an attempt to
predict the loading distribution at the joint will be futile.

The Mechanical Model and Relevant Dynamic Equations

By modeling the body as an ensemble of rigid body segments, the
determination of the resultant loading at a given cross-section of the
body is greatly facilitated. The body can be divided into parts by
imaginary planes passing through the joints under investigation. All
physical connections of one body part with another are then represented
by forces and couples. The calculation of intersegmental loading becomes
straightforward provided that the external loading on the body segments,
the segment inertial properties, and their spatial configurations are
known.

Any body segment taken into consideration may have physical
interactions with the environment. If this is the case, then this
interaction is represented using resultant (external reaction) forces and
couples. These environmental interactions include, for example,
foot-to-floor interaction during gait. Suitable load transducers are

utilized to detect the loads transmitted to the body from the environment. All of these force actions are usually referred to as external forces and couples.

So far, a mechanical model of a linkage of physically-united rigid segments has been made, of which the mechanical interactions with surrounding bodies are represented by forces and couples. In order to proceed with the analysis of the mechanics of the model, other properties, namely, positional and inertial, must be associated with the model.

The positional properties convey the information needed to locate, at any instant in time, the position of any point in a segment relative to an arbitrarily chosen reference observer. This is achieved by defining a local coordinate system (x,y,z) fixed to the moving segment and a global coordinate system (X,Y,Z) fixed to the observer. Given the position vector $\underline{p}$ of any point in the local coordinate system (l.c.s.), the relevant position vector $\underline{P}$ in the global coordinate system (g.c.s.) is given by

$$\underline{P} = [A]\underline{p} + \underline{P}_o \qquad (1)$$

where $[A]$ is the rotation matrix and $\underline{P}_o$ is the position vector of the l.c.s. origin relative to the g.c.s. The columns of matrix $[A]$ are the direction cosines of the l.c.s. axes with respect to the g.c.s. axes.

The inertial properties associated with each model segment are represented by the following parameters of the relevant body segment:

a) mass (m)

b) position vector of the center of mass (CM) in the l.c.s. $(\underline{p}_g)$,

c) principal axes of inertia defined relative to the l.c.s. by the columns of a rotation matrix $[B]$, and

d) moments of inertia about the principal axes passing through the CM (I_x, I_y, I_z).

The above positional and inertial properties thoroughly define the mechanical model. The next step is to determine the equations relating all of the quantities which describe the mechanical behavior of the free-body diagram of the body portion under investigation and, in particular, permit the intersegmental force and couple vectors to be calculated.

Figure la depicts a general free-body diagram consisting of n segments. Point R_s is an arbitrary point at which an external reaction force and couple acting on the s-th segment is applied, while point Q is an arbitrary point to which the intersegmental forces have been reduced. The dynamical equilibrium of the free body requires that the following

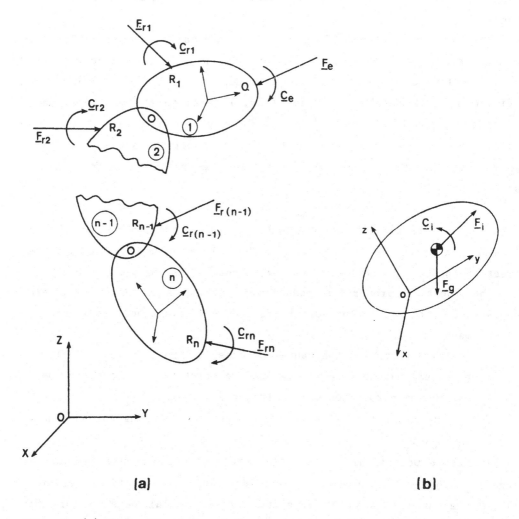

(a)   (b)

Fig. 1 (a) Generalized free-body diagram, and (b) a single segment.

system of equations be satisfied

$$\underline{F}_g + \underline{F}_i + \underline{F}_r + \underline{F}_e = 0 \tag{2}$$
$$\underline{M}_g + \underline{M}_i + \underline{M}_r + \underline{C}_i + \underline{C}_r + \underline{C}_e = 0 \tag{3}$$

where $\underline{F}_g$, $\underline{F}_i$, $\underline{F}_r$, $\underline{C}_i$, and $\underline{C}_r$ are the resultant vectors of the gravitational, inertial, and external reaction forces, and the inertial and external reaction couples acting on the n segments, respectively. $\underline{M}_g$, $\underline{M}_i$, and $\underline{M}_r$ are, respectively, the resultant moment vectors of the gravitational, inertial, and reaction forces acting on the n segments calculated with respect to point Q. $\underline{F}_e$ and $\underline{C}_e$ are the intersegmental force and couple vectors.

Taking into consideration an individual segment (Fig. 1b), the gravitational and inertial force vectors referenced to the g.c.s. acting on the segment are given by the following equations:

$$\underline{F}_g = m \begin{Bmatrix} 0 \\ 0 \\ -g \end{Bmatrix}, \text{ and } \underline{F}_i = -m\ddot{\underline{P}}_g \tag{4},(5)$$

where $\underline{P}_g = [A]\underline{p}_g + \underline{P}_o$.
The inertial couple vector, referenced to the g.c.s. is given by

$$\underline{C}_i = -[A][B] \begin{bmatrix} I_x \dot{\omega}_x + (I_z - I_y) \omega_y \omega_z \\ I_y \dot{\omega}_y + (I_x - I_z) \omega_x \omega_z \\ I_z \dot{\omega}_z + (I_y - I_x) \omega_x \omega_y \end{bmatrix} \tag{6}$$

where

$$\omega_x, \omega_y \text{ and } \omega_z$$

are the segment angular velocity vector components relative to the principal axes of inertia. These can be expressed in terms of angular velocity components in the l.c.s. as:

$$\begin{Bmatrix} \omega_x \\ \omega_y \\ \omega_z \end{Bmatrix} = [B]^T \begin{Bmatrix} \omega_x' \\ \omega_y' \\ \omega_z' \end{Bmatrix} \tag{7}$$

where,

$$\omega_x' = \dot{a}_{12}a_{13} + \dot{a}_{22}a_{23} + \dot{a}_{32}a_{33}, \tag{8}$$

$$\omega_y' = \dot{a}_{13}a_{11} + \dot{a}_{23}a_{21} + \dot{a}_{33}a_{31}, \text{ and} \tag{9}$$

$$\omega_z' = \dot{a}_{11}a_{12} + \dot{a}_{21}a_{22} + \dot{a}_{31}a_{32} \tag{10}$$

where, a_{ij} and $\dot{a}_{ij}$ are the elements of the matrix [A] and its time derivatives, respectively.

The global position vectors of points Q and R_s (s=1,...,n) are also needed for the calculation of $\underline{M}_g$, $\underline{M}_i$, and $\underline{M}_r$. The former position vector is usually given in the l.c.s. and transformed in the g.c.s. using Equation 1. The position vectors of points R_s are usually directly given in the g.c.s.

If the time functions of the positional variables ($\underline{P}_o$, [A]), the inertial parameters (m, $\underline{p}_g$, [B], I_x, I_y, I_z), and the external reaction vectors $\underline{P}_R$, $\underline{F}_r$, and $\underline{C}_r$ are given for each model segment in addition to the local position vector $\underline{p}_Q$, then the intersegmental force and couple vectors can be calculated using the equations given above. In many cases only one external reaction force vector and one external reaction couple vector are required in the model. An example of this would be a force platform measuring the foot-to-floor reactions during gait. In such cases, it is a practical convenience to consider the most distal segment (i.e. segment where external reactions are known) first and progress proximally from segement to segment until all the desired intersegmental forces and couples are known.

The description of the intervening joint kinematics can be obtained from the relative positional information of adjacent body segments. The screw axis of motion is an effective means for such a description. The six parameters which describe the screw axis in each instant of time can be calculated using the time functions of $\underline{P}_o$ and [A] associated with any two segments. Kinzel et al.[1] and Panjabi et al.[2], among others, provide relevant equations.

In the following sections, the experimental methods used to determine the above-mentioned segmental positional variables and inertial parameters are discussed. Various random measurement errors are introduced while measuring the kinematic variables. Therefore, appropriate techniques used for the calculation of the first and second derivatives in Equations 5-10 are also going to be discussed.

Motion Measurement

The motions of the segments which compose the body segment model can be determined in many ways. The following presentation presents the most common schemes for measuring these motions. Space does not allow for a detailed discussion of each method here, so they are simply mentioned briefly and further references are supplied. The motion measurement methods discussed are stereometry, exoskeltal linkages, and accelerometry.

Stereometry permits the three-dimensional (3-D) reconstruction of the instantaneous position of a moving point in a laboratory (global) coordinate system. If at least three noncolinear points fixed in a rigid segement are known, then the position vector and the rotation matrix of this segment can be derived through simple vector calculations, thus fulfilling a basic experimental need.

Stereophotogrammetry, light scanning, and stereosonic systems are techniques using basic concepts of sterometry. All of these entail that the target points be represented by convenient markers, the physical realization of which depends on the particular technique used. In the present context, the target points are anatomical landmarks, or rigid extensions of them, selected according to practical considerations, which include: a) the distances between markers should be sufficiently large for the error propagation from measured marker coordinates to rotation matrix to be minimal, and b) if skin markers are used, relative movement between markers and underlying bone due to soft tissue deformation should be minimal, thus consistent with the assumption of rigidity of the body segment.

Close-range photogrammetry permits the achievement of the present experimental objective with an accuracy that is adequate for most gross body movement analyses. It entails the reconstruction of the 3-D coordinates of a target point with respect to a laboratory coordinate system (object space) from the coordinates of the projections of the point onto at least two planes (image spaces). The images may be obtained from central projections of the object space onto a light-sensitive image plane through a.system of lenses.

Three methods for obtaining photogrammetric measurements are photography, opto-electronic devices, and X-rays. Classical techniques for obtaining protogrammetric measurements use either still of cine photographic cameras[3-5]. Two (or more) still cameras with either stationary or continuously moving film[6,7], or two synchronized cine cameras can be used. A single camera can also be used whereby multiple perspective views are provided by mirrors[4,8]. The markers which designate the anatomical landmark to be tracked may be passive markers of a color in contrast with the background if cine cameras are used, or active light-emitting diodes (LEDs) if still cameras are used. Reflective dots illuminated with a strobe light may also be used instead of LEDs. The marker image coordinates must be digitized prior to further processing.

In recent years great effort has been devoted to technolgical improvements connected with stereophotogrammetry in the field of biomechanics. New optoelectronic devices have been developed as alternatives to the conventional photographic cameras, permitting a direct feeding of the point projection information to a digital computer. The operator time required for data reduction from target point projections can be reduced by an order of magnitude, thus overcoming the major shortcomings of conventional photogrammetry. There are several commercially available optoelectronic motion measurement devices. These devices have different spatial resolutions and sampling frequencies, require different marker types, and allow for various maximum number of markers. The various systems all have advantages and disadvantages and thus selection of a device depends greatly on the needs of the investigator (see References 9-14).

When accurate quantitative knowledge about the relative motion of two opposing bones is required, Roentgenstereophotogrammetry may be used. Based on the same principles as conventional photogrammetry, this technique permits the tracking of the motion of radio-opaque markers, which are usually embedded in the bone, with respect to a fixed reference frame through two X-ray projections[15]. This intrinsically invasive technique represents a health hazard, thus its use is normally limited to cadaver specimens.

Once the image coordinates of the markers are fed to the computer, either through manual digitization of photographs or automatically using opto-electronic devices, the reconstruction of the relevant object space coordinates must be carried out. This triangulation is done through mathematical models (photogrammetric models). Analytical photogrammetry has received renewed attention in recent years among biomechanicians as a consequence of the technological achievements illustrated above[16-23]. Some type of calibration scheme must be incorporated into any photogrammetric model to obtain the 3-D coordinates of a point in observation area. The information needed for the system calibration calculations is provided by a control point distribution, i.e. calibration object, placed within the observation area. The amount of absolute information needed about the geometry of this object differs for different calibration procedures[24-26].

The choice of the position and orientation of the two cameras in relation to each other and with respect to the measurement field is important. Minimum error propagation to the reconstructed target point position is achieved when the cameras are set-up orthogonal to one another and when the distances from the cameras to the target point is a minimum. From practical considerations, however, these conditions cannot always be achieved. The following other factors are to be taken into account:

   a) size of the measurement field and overlap area of the fields of view of the two cameras

   b) size of the cone of light emission of reflection of the markers, and

   c) shadowing by other body segments.

A second method of stereometry involves the use of light-scanning systems. In these systems, three beams of light are swept across the field of view by three multifaceted polygonal mirrors. Two of the mirrors rotate about parallel axes and the third about an axis orthogonal to the others. The markers, small passive pyramidal prisms, reflect light back to the scanner unit where it is detected by photodiodes. The duration to the return of the light pulse is related to the marker position. Identification of individual markers is achieved by their distinct colors. Such systems are reported to exhibit outstanding features, although reports on their evaluation in actual biomechanical applications are not yet available[27].

The final stereometrical methods of position determination discussed are the stereosonic systems. One stereosonic system described by Brumbaugh et al.[28] uses ultrasonic acoustic transmitters to mark anatomical landmarks. Three mutually-orthogonal microphones detect time-multiplexed pulses, from the transmitters, which can be used to deduce marker position based on time delay. This type of system has a small resolution, however, it also has a limited measurement field (only up to $1.0m^3$).

Henning and Nicol[29] describe a stereosonic system based on the Doppler-effect. The marker transmitters emit a fixed-frequency sound. The variations in frequency as detected by a fixed microphone indicate the relative velocity between the marker and microphone to within 0.5%.

If only a measurement of the gross relative motion between adjacent body segments is desired, then exoskeletal linkage systems can be used.

By externally attaching these linkages to the body segments, the relevant angular and linear positions can be measured, usually using potentiometers. Planar, triaxial, and six-degree-of-freedom spatial devices have been developed using several electro-mechanical techniques[2,30-33]. If joint kinematics are of interest, the device should be attached directly to the opposing bones, which restricts this type of experimental approach to in-vitro situations[2,34]. Since the position data provided by electro-mechanical transducers are relative in nature, they do not, in general, serve the purpose of determining the intersegmental actions.

Accelerometers can be used to completely describe the motion of a rigid body as velocity and displacement information can be derived through integration and known initial conditions[35]. Accelerometers and their related wiring are often bulky and may encumber the subject. Acceleration data acquisition and reduction is quite demanding because of the large number of quantities that have to be measured. Technical problems arise when regarding the determination of the initial conditions. Due to these facts, accelerometry does not seem to be competitive with the other methods discussed for determining body segment kinematics. Accelerometry does play a fundamental role in joint biomechanics in instances when the body segments are subjected to either high frequency vibrations or impulsive external forces[36].

Body Segment Inertial Parameters

The determination of subject-specific segemental inertial parameter values to be assigned to the relevant mechanical model segments is another important problem in the biomechanics of human movement. Current methods for the in-vivo experimental assessment of those parameters are complex, and some of them (eg. gamma scanning methods) may be harmful to the subjects health. Therefore, the use of these experimental assessments for routine analysis is debatable.

Instead, prediction techniques, which compute the inertial parameters from anthropometric dimensions, are usually preferred. Due to space limitations, individual discussions of the many prediction techniques reported is not warranted here. Rather, references will be provided for the interested reader. Two major prediction technique methodologies can be classified. One deals with estimation through regression equations, and the other estimation using geometrical approximations.

The regression equations have been determined through statistical analysis of data obtained from sample populations of subjects. Measurements have been made using cadaver specimens[3,37-42] and living subjects[4,43,44]. These regression equations generally involve functions of body weight, stature, segment lengths and circumferences, or other easily measurable quantities from which the inertia properties can be deduced.

The geometrical approximation method has been used by several investigators, with the most thorough studies having been performed by Hanavan[45], Jensen[46], and Hatze[47]. This method, in general, provides a means of representing the irregular shapes of the different body segments with standard geometric forms which are capable of simple mathematical description.

In practice, decisions as to which method or methods are to be used to predict inertial parameters must be made. Several investigators have performed checks on the methods discussed above and made suggestions as to the accuracies of them[48,49,50].

Numerical Differentiation Techniques

It is a basic interest to the biomechanical analyst to obtain good estimates of human displacement data, together with their first and second derivatives. Errors in this data will be directly translated to errors in the segment inertial force and moment calculations. Numerical differentiation of the relevant experimental data, which are affected by relatively large experimental errors, especially when stereometric techniques are used, may easily lead to unstable solutions. Appropriate information retrieval procedures must be applied as well as a wise choice of the motion data sampling frequency in order to alleviate some of the difficulties associated with differentiation.

Spurious wild points in the data, and occasional occlusion of markers, must be corrected prior to any subsequent analysis. Systematic errors, caused by such things as skin marker or exoskeletal structures, are difficult to eliminate from the acquired data but may be minimized by proper equipment design. Various random errors also occur due to effects occurring within the image-processing equipment and digitization of the marker coordinates. These random errors are usually of high frequency content, rendering the direct use of raw experimental data in calculations which entail time differentiation impossible. Classical numerical differentiation procedures may lead to unstable numerical processes. Solving this typical problem in experimental biomechanics is critical.

Several investigators have evaluated numerical differentiation procedures and have provided methods of determining the precision of differentiation techniques[52-54]. The proper choice of the motion data sampling frequency is of crucial importance. The best possible signal and noise description requires a high sampling frequency, while computer memory and running time limitations dictate a low sampling frequency. A compromising sampling frequency value must be sought.

All of the numerical differentiation techniques developed can be grouped into one of two categories. Time domain techniques[51,53-58] require that the structure of the underlying function be known and a homogeneous set of analytical functions be associated with it. Frequency domain techniques[17,59-66], often referred to as filters, may be divided into two subgroups according to whether or not they require the explicit calculation of the Fourier transform of the data (details in references).

Some of the many differentiation techniques have been evaluated comparatively, but only in a qualitative manner. It is difficult to say, at present, which technique is the "best" for a specific application.

ANATOMICAL JOINT MODELING

Once the resultant intersegmental loading at a joint is known, the much more difficult task of determining how the resultant load is shared by the various structures of that joint must be undertaken. The intersegmental forces and couples at a joint must be balanced by the actions of the musculature, ligaments, and bony structures associated with that joint. The main difficulty arises from the fact that the number of structures which transmit the load is usually far greater than the number of available equilibrium equations. Thus, the problem is indeterminate. The remainder of this section is devoted to discussing some of the analytical modeling necessary to arrive at a reasonable joint model. The following section will then discuss various methods of predicting solutions to this problem while presenting several simple examples illustrating various solution possibilities.

Coordinate System Selection

The selection of a coordinate system is very important in the development of an analytical joint model. It is usually quite useful to align a Cartesian coordinate system along some preferred anatomical axis. For example, in the case of the elbow joint (Fig. 2) a good selection of axes would have one axis (X-axis in this case) correspond with the elbow flexion-extension axis. This coordinate system selection is useful because it is desirable to have an axis about which primarily muscles contribute to the moment. This allows solving for muscle forces independent of the other structures.

Equilibrium Equations

Before the equilibrium equations can be used it is necessary to transform, via suitable transformation matrices, the intersegemental forces and couples (moments) to the joint axes coordinate system. In many cases the body fixed local coordinate systems, as described earlier, can be made to coincide with the joint model coordinate system so that no transformation is necessary.

The equations of equilibrium for any joint can be written as Equations 11 and 12:

$$\underline{F}_e = \sum_{i=1}^{m} \underline{f}_{im} + \sum_{i=1}^{k} \underline{f}_{ik} + \sum_{i=1}^{c} \underline{f}_{ic} \qquad (11)$$

$$\underline{C}_e = \sum_{i=1}^{m} (\underline{r}_{im} \times \underline{f}_{im}) + \sum_{i=1}^{k} (\underline{r}_{ik} \times \underline{f}_{ik}) + \sum_{i=1}^{c} (\underline{r}_{ic} \times \underline{f}_{ic}) \qquad (12)$$

Where $\underline{F}_e$ and $\underline{C}_e$ are the intersegmental resultant force and couple respectively defined at the joint coordinate system origin Q; $\underline{f}_{im}$, $\underline{f}_{ik}$, and $\underline{f}_{ic}$ are respectively the forces in the i-th muscle and ligament, and on the articular surface contact region; $\underline{r}_{im}$, $\underline{r}_{ik}$, and $\underline{r}_{ic}$ are vectors from Q to a point on the line of action of the i-th muscle, ligament, and articular contact force, respectively; m is the number of muscles used in the model, k the number of ligaments, and c the number of simply-connected articular contact regions within the joint; "x" denotes vector cross product.

Equations 11 and 12 result in six equilibrium equations as both equations corresponding to the X, Y, and Z Cartesian coordinate system directions. It should now be apparent that the number of unknowns can greatly outnumber the number of equations.

Anatomical and physiological constraint conditions must also be used to aid in finding a feasible solution to the equilibrium equations. The constraint conditions applicable to all joints include that the tendinous (musculature) and ligamentous structures transmit only tensile loads and that the articulating surfaces transmit only compressive loads. Electromyograhic data, which give an indication of activity in the respective muscles, are sometimes used in the development of a joing model but are more commonly used to validate or dispute a muscle force solution.

Geometric Considerations

Before Equations 11 and 12 can be used, a complete description of the geometry of all the load carrying structures must be made. The lines of action (directions of force vectors) for each muscle, ligament, and

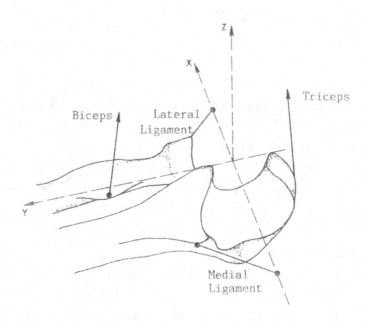

Fig. 2 Plausible selection of axes at the elbow joint.

joint contact force must be determined. A vector from the joint center, the reference location at which the intersegemental resultants are known, to the lines of action of all the force vectors must also be determined. These vectors must all be expressed in the coordinate system being used at the joint of interest. Also, these vectors can change drastically as an exercise is being performed, and therefore must be position dependent to be accurate.

The line of action of some muscles and ligaments, can be taken as a line from the point of origin to the point of insertion. With the muscle (ligament) origin and insertion positions known in the appropriate coordinate system, the line of action of the muscle (ligament) force and the vector from the joint center to the muscle (ligament) can also be determined for different joint position.

Many muscles have tendonious origins and insertions and the determination of the points of attachment is an easy task. This is also the case for many ligaments. Sometimes, however, the determination of a point of muscle or ligament attachment is not a very exact procedure. Some muscles and ligaments have relatively large areas of attachment. In these instances, the investigator must estimate a "good" point of attachment for the structure being modelled. Often, this approximation is taken as the geometric center of the attachment area. The fact that the exact line of action of a muscle or ligament is sometimes not known introduces some error in the joint model.

Modelling of line of action using a straight line, origin to insertion approach is quite acceptable for some structures, such as the lateral collateral ligament of the knee, and not so acceptable for others, such as the biceps brachi. The biceps "bulges" around underlying musculature in most elbow joint positions and rarely, if ever, acts through a straight line.

A better model for the line of action of the biceps (or other non-straight structure) would be a line which passes through the cross-sectional area centroid of the muscle. Attempting to accurately determine the area centroid of a muscle at numerous locations along the

muscle, and for many joint positions is a very laborous undertaking. An
et al.[67] did this by transversely cutting frozen cadaver arms at closely
spaced intervals and calculating the geometric centroids of the muscle.
This procedure worked well in that possible generalizations as to the
locations of the centroids of the muscles crossing the elbow could be
determined for the elbow positions they investigated. (Six different
elbow positions were studied.) However, an infinite combination of elbow
flexion-extension and forearm supination-pronation positions exists.
Obviously, to arrive at a relatively useful position dependent centroid
line of action model for a muscle or ligament many man hours will likely
be needed.

To avoid trying to measure the centroid of a muscle or ligament,
various lines of actions may be modeled as arcs of constant curvature or
as pulley and cable systems. The line of action of the gluteous
maximums, for example, acts along an arc of fairly fixed curvature and at
a roughly fixed distance from the hip joint center. Many joint extensor
muscles, the triceps for example, act as cables going over pulleys of
fixed radius when the joint, the elbow in this case, is considerably
flexed. The line of action of the muscle acts tangential to the
imaginary pulley. This pulley-cable model may work quite well for some
joint positions, but a different model may have to be used for other
positions.

It is necessary to clarify what is meant by articulating joint
contact force used in Equations 11 and 12. When two articulating joint
surfaces are forced together a compressive stress over some area exists.
Generally, joint surfaces are covered with cartilage which acts to
distribute the load. However, when the joint model is made it is
convenient to replace the joint stress acting on an area with a joint
force acting at a point. The point of application of this force is
considered to be the center of pressure.

An analysis of the rigid body geometry of the joint surfaces is
useful in determining the direction of a joint contact force. As the
coefficient of friction on the joint surface is normally negligibly

small, the joint force can be taken as acting normal to the joint surface.

The geometry of most joint surfaces is fairly complex and varies among individuals. Extensive studies have been performed to accurately measure and define joint surface geometries. However, most investigators choose definable geometric shapes such as cones, arches, and hemispheres to model joint surfaces. The geometry of the joint surface also fixes the solution space for the joint contact forces. The joint contact force must have its point of application within the area defining the joint surface.

Modelling the lines of action for all the muscle, ligament, and contact forces included in a dynamic joint model is a very complex task. The locations, as well as the directions, of all of these force vectors must be determined in the joint coordinate system. Any combination of the muscle and ligament line of action models discussed, as well as others, could be used depending on the structure of interest and the joint position. It is also necessary to model the geometry of the joint surface, be it by accurate measurement or suitable geometric shape approximation.

CALCULATION OF MUSCLE AND JOINT FORCES

Once the intersegmental resultant forces and moments have been determined and a suitable joint model devised, the problem of distributing these forces and moments between the different joint structures is at hand. The equilibrium equations for any anatomical joint (Equations 11 and 12) must be satisfied, while at the same time the solutions for the magnitudes of the loads carried by the various joint structures must be within certain physiologically possible ranges. Due to complexity of the joints of the human body the equilibrium equations contain many more unknown values than there are equations describing joint behavior. Thus, most distribution problems are highly indeterminate.

Solution Methods Without Using Optimization

Various analytical methods are used to arrive at reasonable
predictions for the load distribution between the various structures
which satisfy the equilibrium equations. Equations 11 and 12 can be
solved uniquely if the joint model can be simplified to include only as
many load carrying joint structures as there are equations. Thus,
solutions to be indeterminate problem can be found by anatomical or
functional simplifications[68-76]. Muscles with similar function and
structure can be grouped together to simplify the model.
Electromyographic (EMG) dignals which indicate muscle activity can also
aid in the decision of when to exclude or include various muscles from
the model[77,78]. In many activities the ligaments associated with the
joint of interest can be assumed not to be taut. Since ligaments can not
carry compressive forces, these ligamentous structures can be neglected
in the joint model thus simplifying the analysis.

Many possible solutions exist for Equations 11 and 12 depending on
which structures are included in the joint model. Some of the possible
solutions, however, result in inadmissable solutions. Inadmissable
solutions occur if a muscle or ligament force is calculated to be
compressive or a joint force is calculated to be tensile. Also,
physiologically unacceptable stresses in a structure mean that solution
is not feasible. By including different structures in the simplified
joint model, in a trial-and-error basis, it is usually possible to
bracket an acceptable range for the loading in any particular structure.

Consider, for example, a static (90° flexion), two-dimensional, one
degree-of-freedom, model of the elbow joint (Fig. 3). Three muscles; the
biceps, brachioradialis, and brachialis, and two rigid links, connected
by a frictionless pin joint, are included in the joint model. Assume
negligible link mass and consider a resultant external couple of 20Nm in
the direction shown. Assume that no anatagonist muscle activity and no
ligament loading occur, indicating that the three muscle tensions must
somehow balance the resultant moment.

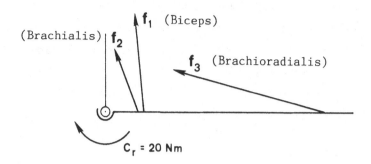

Fig. 3 Simplified Elbow Joint Model

The equilibrium moment equations (Eqn. 12) reduce to one equation in three unknowns; the force in the biceps, f_1, the force in the brachialis, f_2, and the force in the brachioradialis, f_3. The resulting equilibrium moment equation can be written as:

External Couple $= r_1 f_1 + r_2 f_2 + r_3 f_3 = 20$ Nm.   (13)

Where r_1, r_2, and r_3 correspond to the moment arms of the biceps, brachialis, and brachioradialis, respectively. An et.al.[79] give values for elbow flexion-extension moment arms of various upper limb muscles. These values were determined using serial cross-sectional anatomical analysis and are given in Table 1. Also given are the physiological cross sectional areas (PCSA) of the three muscles, as reported by An, et.al. and defined as the muscle volume divided by the true muscle fiber length at the resting position.

Even with all of the simplifications made to arrive at this model, the equation defining the systems behavior is still indeterminate and an infinite number of possible solutions exist. It is not the authors' intent to determine a best solution to the problem at hand or to even suggest that this simple a model even accurately simulates actual elbow joint behavior. However, this model can be used to illustrate many of the approaches used to solve the indeterminate problem.

By including only one muscle in the model a unique solution can be obtained. Including only the biceps (f_2 and f_3 zero), Equation 13 can be used to solve for the biceps tension.

$$f_1 = \frac{\text{External Couple}}{r_1} = \frac{20}{0.046} = 435N \qquad\qquad (14)$$

Similary, if only the brachialis or only the brachioradialis are used in the model, values of f_2 equal 588N and f_3 equal 367N can be computed for the single muscle models. (Table 2 shows a summary of possible muscle force solutions to this problem for each solution method discussed.) Although all three of these solutions satisfy equilibrium, they are unrealistic in that EMG studies for such a loading indicate activity in all three of these elbow flexors[77,80]. In this oversimplified model limiting the number of unknowns to the number of equations does not provide exceptable solutions. However, in more complex three dimensional joint models this approach can provide useful information.

TABLE 1:   Elbow flexor moment arms, r_i, at 90 degree flexion, and physiological cross sectional areas ($PCSA_i$) of the Biceps, Brachialis, and Brachioradiolis.

i	Muscle	r_i(cm)	$PCSA_i$(cm^2)
1	Biceps	4.6	4.6
2	Brachialis	3.4	7.0
3	Brachioradialis	7.5	1.5

With the muscle forces known, the joint reaction forces can be computed by satisfying the force equilibrium equations. Equations 11 can be written, in this example, as:

$$\underline{F}_e = \sum_{i=1}^{3} (\underline{f}_{im}) + \underline{f}_c = 0.$$ (15)

In this example, using a pin joint assumption for the elbow joint, the single joint contact force simply acts through the joint center and balances the muscle force in horizontal and vertical directions.

In a more realistic model of joint geometry, the joint contact forces may act at several locations within the joint[73,81]. For instance, a realistic three dimensional model of the elbow joint would likely include several humeral-ulmar joint force contact areas as well as a humeral-radial joint force contact region. With an inclusion of a more complex joint geometry, and possibly several ligament force unknowns, these simplification approaches to the indeterminate problem become more difficult to solve and optimization approaches, to be discussed later, may be more desirable.

An alternate method of solution, which distributes equal stresses amoung all three muscles, is to impose proportial load sharing amoung the muscles based on their physiological cross sectional areas[82-84]. Applying this idea to the elbow joint problem results in the following:

$$f_i = \frac{PCSA_1}{PCSA_{max}} f_{max}$$ (16)

Where, $PCSA_{max}$ = PCSA of largest muscle = $PCSA_2$ = 7.0 cm^2

and f_{max} = Force in largest PCSA muscle = f_2. Then f_1 and f_2 become:

$$f_1 = \frac{4.6}{7.0} f_2 \qquad f_3 = \frac{1.5}{7.0} f_2$$ (17)

Now, using the equilibrium equations (Eqn 13) to get;

$$20 \text{ Nm} = r_1 f_1 + r_2 f_2 + r_3 f_3$$

$$= 0.046 \frac{4.6}{7.0} f_2 + 0.034 \; f_2 + 0.075 \frac{1.5}{7.0} f_2 \qquad (18)$$

results in:

$$f_1 = 164 \text{ N} \qquad f_2 = 249 \text{ N} \qquad f_3 = 53 \text{ N}$$

Using this method of solution results in equal stresses developed in all of the muscles. The muscle stress, simply defined as the muscle force divided by the muscle PCSA, developed in the three muscles in this case is 356 kPa. This stress level is within the maximum permissable muscle stress levels found in the literature[85]. (A value of about 600 kPa for the maximum isometric muscle stress is generally accepted).

The hypothesis, that the muscles are equally stressed, used in this approach is most suited to cases where the muscles approach their maximum strength[83]. This hypothesis will not hold for lightly loaded situations, as likely not as many muscles will be activated in such a case.

Load sharing between muscles proportional to their masses has also been used[86,87]. For example, the tension in the biceps and brachialis can be taken equal while the tension in the brachioradialis would be half the tension in the biceps[88]. This results in the following muscle forces:

$$f_1 = f_2 = 170 \text{ N} \qquad f_3 = 85 \text{ N}$$

By prescribing suitable proportional ratios among the muscle forces in a model, a solution to the indeterminate problem can often be found. Although this approach is dependent on the judgement of the investigator, it provides an order of magnitude estimation to the force distribution, which generally relates well temporally with EMG signals. EMG validation is generally an ultimate factor used to determine the feasibility of a muscle force solution, regardless of the solution method used.

Solution methods Using Optimization Techniques

Methods of solving the indeterminate Equations 11 and 12 without significant simplification of the functional anatomy involve seeking an optimum solution which minimizes or maximizes some process or action. With the advent of high speed computers, optiminzation procedures, which require many iterations of equation solving to evenually find an optimal solution, have developed rapidly. Optimization techniques of solution allow for the inclusion of more unknowns in the joint model, thus permitting a more realistic model to be made. Many muscle force solutions obtained using optimization correlate well with EMG patterns, thus indicating reasonable estimates of joint loading.

Optimization methods of solution are significantly more involved than those previously described. In this approach, some value, say U, which is defined as a function of the variables to be determined, is maximized or minimized within bounds established by the constraints imposed on the variables.

Although the use of optimization techniques is widely established in biomechanic studies, the selection of an optimization or cost function, U, is still open to discussion. The selection of an optimization function depends on the activity being performed. It may be warranted to minimize joint contact forces, when modelling a joint with degenerative joint disease, in an attempt to minimize pain. Minimizing fatigue might work well in some instances but would be unreasonable for analyzing short-term activities. Various researchers have utilized different optimization functions with varying degrees of success. The following will review some of these attempts at solving the problem of muscle activity. Several optimization method solutions of the three muscle elbow joint model (Fig. 3) will also be presented.

Optimization techniques can generally be categorized as linear or nonlinear depending on the form of the optimization function. If a linear function is to be optimized, a unique minimum and maximum always occur within the solution space bounded by the constrait conditions. If a nonlinear function is to be optimized, finding an extremum in the solution space is a more difficult task. Often, several local mixima or minima occur in the solution space. Care must be taken not to mistakenly accept any local extremum as the extremum for the entire solution space (global extremum). Various programming schemes must be used to ensure that the correct optimum is found. It is also possible, with a nonlinear cost function, to have two or more equal optimum values in the same solution space. The extra difficulties associated with nonlinear as compared to linear optimization techniques have led most researchers to develop linear optimization functions in their attempts to solve the indeterminate muscle force problem.

Many of the early works dealing with the use of optimization techniques dealt with simply minimizing the sum of the muscle force. Penrod et. al.[89] developed a wrist joint model and Yeo[90] investigated the elbow joint in an attempt to determine, via minimizing the sum of the muscle forces, a solution to the redundant muscle force problem at these respective joints. They both concluded that the muscles with the longest moment arms produce the lowest muscle forces. Minimizing the sum of the muscle forces is a purely geometric optimization, results in very few muscles being predicted active, and does not result in good correlation with EMG activity.

Seireg and Arvikar[91] minimized the sum of all muscle forces plus four times the sum of the moments produced by the muscles of all the joints in the lower extremities. They proposed that this linear criterion suitably controlled the muscle load sharing during static posture and quasi-static locomotion. They predicted few muscles to be active simultaneously and reported that relatively small muscles generated large forces during gait while larger ones generated nearly no force at all. Although this study did not provide great results, it is of importance in that it first demonstrated the use of optimization techniques in solving a complex leg muscle force problem.

Hardt[92] also analyzed the leg during normal human walking using linear optimization methods. To include some of the physiology of the system and the dynamic properties of the muscles, Hardt ultimately settled on an in-depth model of muscle thermodynamics to use as a cost function. This mechanico-chemical energy model depended on the muscle lengths and muscle contractile velocities. As with other researchers, Hardt's data showed some correlation with EMG activity, but some unrealistic muscle forces were predicted.

In an analysis of the finger and thumb joints, Chao and An[93] studied thirty different linear optimization criteria. They minimized such parameters as the sum of muscle forces, the sum of joint contact forces, the weighted sum of muscle forces, and the sum of constraint moments. Only six unqiue sets of optimal solutions were obtained, thus indicating that the majority of the optimal criteria was interrelated.

In the three muscle elbow joint model example, as solution space as shown on Fig. 4 occurs. The planar solution space occurs because the moment equilibrium equation is linear. The solution space represents all possible solutions to the equilibrium equation. The point of the solution on the space is governed by the optimization criteria. If n muscles (unknowns) are modelled the solution space would be a "surface" in n-dimensional space. Minimizing the sum of the muscles, in our elbow model, gives

$$U = \sum_{i=1}^{3} f_i , \qquad\qquad (19)$$

which results in

$$f_1 = 0 \quad f_2 = 0 \quad f_3 = 267 \text{ N}.$$

Only one muscle, the one with the longest moment arm, is predicted to be active. The optimization results in an inadmissibly high muscle force and provides no synergistic muscle activity.

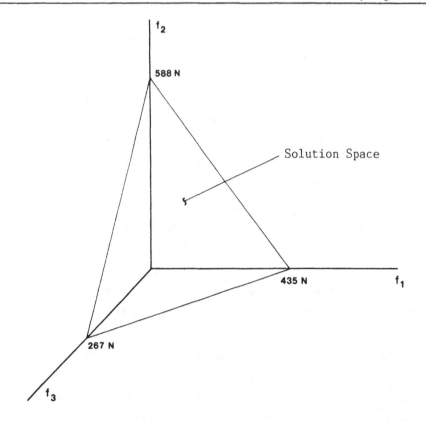

Fig. 4   Solution Space For Three Muscle Elbow Joint Model.

One major limitation with the optimization schemes discussed so far is that no upper bounds were imposed on the muscle forces. Limiting the muscle forces to some maximum prevents inadmissibly high muscle forces from occurring and causes the recruitment of more muscles into the solution.

In an analysis of the elbow joint, Crowninshield[94] applied an upper limit to the muscle stress $(f_1/PCSA_1)$. He used minimization of the sum of the muscle stresses as his optimization function. Crowninshield showed that without imposing the maximum stress limit that the results were not valid. He used a maximum stress value equal to the maximum permissable value found in the literature (600 kPa) and a value below this value as his upper limits to muscle stress. His conclusion was that by imposing maximum stress values below those physically possible a good correlation between muscle force prediction and EMG signals can be obtained for the activities he studied. He also commented that optimization techniques which impose the maximum physiological stress limit are reasonable for only very strenuous activities, and that in most instances this limit should be considerably reduced.

The idea of limiting muscle stress (or force) can be further illustrated through our elbow model example. Minimizing the sum of the muscle stress results in the following cost function.

$$U = \sum_{i=1}^{3} (f_i/PCSA_i) \qquad (20)$$

Without imposing any upper limits on the muscle stresses the results would be

$$f_1 = 0 \qquad f_2 = 588 \text{ N} \qquad f_3 = 0.$$

Here, the brachialis is utilized in preference to the other muscles because it has the largest product of PCSA and moment arm. This solution is not acceptable however for reasons mentioned previously.

Imposing a miximum allowable stress limit equal to the maximum physiologically achievable muscle stress, 600 kPa, reduces the solutions space to that shown in Fig. 5. This imposition rules out excessively high muscle stresses. Using the cost function of Equation 20, along with the imposed upper limits on the muscle stresses, which can be written in terms of limits on the muscle forces as

$$f_i \leqslant (PCSA_i)(600 \text{ kPa}), \qquad (21)$$

results in

$$f_1 = 124 \text{ N} \qquad f_2 = 420 \text{ N} \qquad f_3 = 0.$$

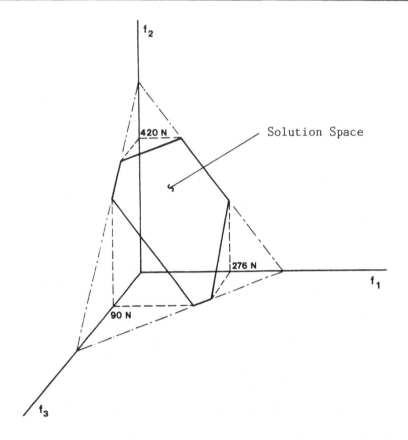

Fig. 5   Solution Space with Upper Stress Limit of 600 kPa Imposed as
         Constraint.

This indicates that the brachialis, f_2, is employed to its fullest extent
and that the biceps, f_1, is required to help balance the external moment.
This is not likely the case when such a moderate task is being performed
(i.e. opposing a 20 Nm moment).   Only during an extremely strenuous
activity would a muscle be so highly stressed.

    Reducing the imposed limit on the muscle stress further reduces the
solution space and will not allow muscles to be stressed to their
physiological limits.   It was shown earlier that setting the muscle
forces proportional to their PCSA resulted in an equal stress
distribution among the muscles equal to 356 kPa.   This value indicates

the minimum value that could be used for the maximum stress limit which would still result in a solution. Using a value above this value and below 600 kPa would be most plausible when simulating actual moderate activity. Imposing a maximum stress limit of 400 kPa results in

$$f_1 = 184 \text{ N} \quad f_2 = 280 \text{ N} \quad f_3 = 27 \text{ N}.$$

This particular scheme indicates activity in all three muscles and produces muscle stress magnitudes well within physiological bounds.

Pedotti et. al.[95] used another criterion to impose upper limits on the muscle forces. They calculated a maximum possible force, f_{max}, for each muscle for each instant of time during human gait. They based this calculation on the instantaneous muscle length and muscle velocity of shortening. Pedotti et. al. studied two linear optimization functions,

$$U_1 = \sum f_i \qquad \text{and} \qquad U_2 = \sum f_i / f_{maxi} \tag{22}$$

and two nonlinear functions,

$$U_3 = \sum f_i^2 \quad \text{and} \quad U_4 = \sum (f_i / f_{maxi})^2. \tag{23}$$

The method of Lagrange multipliers was used to perform the nonlinear optimization. Based on a correlation of predicted muscle forces with reported EMG activity, they claimed a preference for U_4 as an optimization criteria.

Patriarco et.al.[96] reevaluated the works done by Seireg and Arvikar[91] and Hardt[92]. They implemented limits on the muscle load levels based on restricting similar muscles to share the load in proportion to their cross-sectional areas, and based on the criteria proposed by Pedotti et. al.[95]. Their results indicate that the "addition of physiologically-based constraints are essential to distinguishing the role of individual muscles". A relative insensitivity to variations in the optimization schemes (minimizing muscle force[91] as opposed to minimizing mechanico-chemical energy[92] was reported, although significant variations were realized by lowering the limits on the ·muscle load levels.

Crowninshield and Brand[97] predicted muscle activity based on a criterion of maximum endurance of musculoskeletal function. Based on the inversely nonlinear relationship between muscle force and muscle contraction endurance[98,99] they proposed a cost function of

$$U = \sum_i (f_i/PCSA_i)^3. \tag{24}$$

This scheme tends to keep individual muscle stresses low, predicts force activity in numerous muscles, and achieves maximum endurance of activity as defined in the literature. When applied to human walking this scheme provides good results, as claimed for prolonged or repetitive activities.

Applying this nonlinear cost function, Equation 24, to the elbow joint example, and using Lagrange multipliers to facilitate the optimization, the following muscle forces can be computed:

$$f_1 = 168 \text{ N} \qquad f_2 = 272 \text{ N} \qquad f_3 = 40 \text{ N}$$

So, as prophisied by Crowninshield and Brand[97], the muscle stresses are low and all of the muscles are active.

Another optimization technique used to solve the indeterminate problem of predicting muscle and joint forces was presented by An et.al.[79]. They introduced additional inequality conditions dealing with muscle stress, namely,

$$f_i/PCSA_i \leq \sigma. \tag{25}$$

The variable σ represents the upper bound for all muscle stresses. Their optimization involved minimizing σ. The cost function can be written as

$$U = \sigma \tag{26}$$

This method of solution requires only linear programming and is claimed to compare favorably with minimizing the summation of the square of muscle stress.

Employing the method of An et. al.[79] to solve the example problem results in

$$f_1 = 164 \text{ N} \qquad f_2 = 249 \text{ N} \qquad f_3 = 53 \text{ N}.$$

Note that for a distribution of muscle forces based on only one equation that this solution is the same solution that was obtained by setting the muscle forces proportional to the muscle cross sectional areas, and it results in equal muscle stresses for all three muscles. However, this is not the case when more than one equation is used for distributing muscle forces.

Recently, Cope[100] completed a meticulous study in determining leg muscle forces during human gait. He imposed physiological maximum and minimum force limitations for each muscle based on the muscle's instantaneous length, instantaneous velocity, cross-sectional area, and rest length. Two different, physiologically based, cost functions were investigated with the results showing surprisingly few differences, and close agreement with the phasing of EMG activity.

In summary, Table 2 indicates some of the infinite number of mathermatically possible muscle force solutions to a simple one degree of freedom elbow joint model. However, not all mathematical solutions are physiologically acceptable. Of the physiologically acceptable solutions, the one which provides the best correlation of muscle force prediction with EMG patterns for the same activity will most likely indicate the best muscle force prediction solution. The selection of a solution scheme rests with the researcher and depends on the joint being modelled, the activity being preformed, and the degree of complexity and accuracy the researcher deems necessary for an acceptable muscle and joint force solution.

Table 2: Muscle force solutions for the simplified elbow model using different constraint conditions.

| | | Force, N | | |
		f_1	f_2	f_3
1.	Single Muscle Models			
	1.1 Biceps, f_1	435	0	0
	1.2 Brachialis, f_2	0	588	0
	1.3 Brachioradialis, f_3	0	0	267
2.	Muscle force proportional to cross-sectional area	164	249	53
3.	Muscle force proportional to muscle mass	170	170	85
4.	Minimize $\sum f_i$	0	0	267
5.	Minimize $\sum (f_i/\text{PCSA}_i)$ such that $0 \leqslant f_i/\text{PCSA}_i \leqslant \sigma$			
	5.1 σ unbounded	0	588	0
	5.2 $\sigma = 600$ kPa	124	420	0
	5.3 $\sigma = 400$ kPa	184	280	27
6.	Minimize $\sum (f_i/\text{PCSA}_i)^3$	168	272	40
7.	Minimize σ	164	249	53

It shall be reiterated that, regardless of the muscle and joint force solution scheme used, the predictions of muscle and joint forces will only be as good as the data used to calculate them. The precision achieved in detemining the external resultant forces and moments can be more influential in predicting accurate muscle and joint forces than the muscle force solution scheme. Thus, scrupulous care must be taken during all aspects of solving the muscle and joint force prediction problem.

REFERENCES

1. Kinzel, G.L., Hall, A.S., Jr. and B.M. Hillberry, Measurement of the Total Motion between Two Body Segments-I. Analytical Development. J. Biomechanics, 5, 93, 1972.

2. Panjabi, M.M., Krag, M.M., and V.K. Goel, A Technique of Measurement and Description of Three-Dimensional Six Degrees-of-Freedom Motion of a Body Joint with an Application of the Human Spine, J. Biomechanics, 14, 447, 1981.

3. Braune, C.W., Fisher, O., and Der Gang des Menschen I., Abb. Math. Phys. Cl. Kon. Sachs. Ges. Wissensch, 21, 151, 1895.

4. Bernstein, N.A. The Coordination and Regulation of Movements, Pergamon Press Ltd., 1967.

5. Marey, E.J. La Methode Graphique dans les Sciences Experimentales, 2nd edition with supplement, le Development de las Methode Graphique par la Photographie, G. Masson, Paris, 1885.

6. Cappozzo, A. Strereophotogrammetric System for Kinesiological Studies, Med. and Biol. Eng. and Comput. 21, 217, 1983.

7. Wyss, U.P. and Pollak, V.A., Kinematic Data Acquisition System for Two or Three-Dimensional Motion Analysis, Med. and Biol. Eng. and Comput., 19, 287, 1981.

8. Morasso, P. and Tagliasco, V., Analysis of Human Movements: Spatial Localization with Multiple Perspective Views, Med. and Biol. Engng. and Comput., 21,74, 1983.

9.   Taylor, K.D., Mottier, F.M., Simmons, D.W., Cohen, W., Pavlack Jr., R., Cornell, P., and Haukins, G.B, An Automated Motion Measurement System for Clinical Gait Analysis, J. Biomechanics, 15, 505, 1982.

10. Winter, D.A., Greenlaw, R.K., and Hobson, D.A., Television-Computer Analysis of Kinematics of Human Gait, Comp. Biomed. Res., 5, 1972.

11. Jarrett, M.O., Andrews, B.J., and Paul, J.P., Quantitative Analysis of Locomotion Using Television, Proc. of ISPO World Congress, Montreaux, Switzerland, 1974.

12. Lindholm, L.E, An Optoelectronic Instrument for Remote On-Line Movement Monitoring, Biomechanics, IV, Nelson, R.C. and Morehouse, C.A., Eds., University Park Press, Baltimore, 510, 1974.

13. Leo, T. and Macellari, V., On Line Microcomputer System for Gait Analysis Data Acquisition Based on Commercially Available Optoelectronic Devices, in Biomechanics VII-B, Morecki, A., Fidelus, K., Kedzior, K.and Wit, A., Eds., University Park Press, Baltimore, 1981, 163.

14. Macellari, V. CoSTEL: A Computer Peripheral Remote Sensing Device for 3-Dimensional Monitoring of Human Motion, Med. and Biol. Engng. and Comp., 21, 311, 1983.

15. de Lange, A., van Dijk, R., Huiskes, R., Selvik, G., and van Rens, Th. J.G., The Application of Roentgenstereophotogrammetry for Evaluation of Knee-Joint Kinematics in Vitro, Biomechanics: Principles and Applications, Huiskes, R., Van Campen, D., and De Wijn, J., Eds., Martinus Nijhoff Publishers, The Hague, 1982, 177.

16. Ayoub, M.A., Ayoub, M.M. and J.D. Ramsey. A Stereometric System for Measuring Human Motion, Human Factors, 12, 523, 1970.

17. Woltring, H.J. Calibration and Measurement in 3-D Monitoring of Human Motion. II: Experimental Results and Discussion, Biotelemetry, 3, 65, 1976.

18. Shapiro, R, The Direct Linear Transformation Method for Three-Dimensional Cinematography, Res.Q., 49, 197, 1978.

19. Andriacchi, T.P., Hampton, S.J., Shultz, A.B., and Galante, J.O., Three Dimensional Coordinate Data Processing in Human Motion Analysis, J. Biomech. Engng., 101, 279, 1979.

20. Dapena, J., Harman, E.A., and Miller, J.A., Three Dimensional Cinematography with Control Object of Unknown Shape, J. Biomechanics, 15, 11, 1982.

21. Miller, N.R., Shapiro, R., and McLaughlin, T.M., A Technique for Obtaining Spatial Kinematic Parameters of Segments of Biomechanical Systems from Cinematographic Data, J. Biomechanics, 13, 535, 1980.

22. Gosh, S.K. Analytical Photogrammetry.   Pergamon Press Ltd., New York, 1979.

23. Abdel-Aziz, Y.I. and Karara, H.M., Direct Linear Transformation from Comparator Coordinates into Object Space Coordinates in Close Range Photogrammetry, Proceedings of the ASP/UI Symposium on Close Range Photogrammetry, Urbana, Illinois, 1971.

24. Marzan, T. and Karara, H.M., A Computer Program for Direct Linear Transformation of the Colinearity Condition and some Applications of it. Symposium on Close Range Photogrammetric Systems, American Society of Photogrammetry, Falls Church, 420, 1975.

25. Kenefick, J.F., Gyer, M.S., and Harp, B.F., Analytical Self-calibration, Photogramm. Engng., 38, 1117, 1972.

26. Woltring, H.J. Planar Control in Multi-Camera Calibration for 3-D Gait Studies, J. Biomechanics, 13, 39, 1980.

27. Mitchelson, D., Recording of Movement Without Photography, Techniques for the Analysis of Human Movement, Grieve, D.W., Miller, D., Mitchelson, D., Paul, J.P., and Smith, A.J.,Eds., Lepus Books: London, 1975.

28. Brumbaugh, R.B., Crowninshield, R.D., Blair, W.F. and Andrews, J.G., An In-vivo Study of Normal Wrist Kinematics, J. Biomech. Engng., 104, 176, 1982.

29. Hennig, E.M. and Nicol, K., Velocity Measurement without Contact on Body Surface Points by Means of the Acoustical Doppler Effect,

Biomechanics V-B, Komi, P.V., Ed., University Park Press, Baltimore, 1976, 449.

30. Chao, E.Y., Justification of Triaxial Goniometer for the Measurement of Joint Rotation, J. Biomechanics, 13, 989, 1980.

31. Johnston, R.C. and Smidt, G.L., Measurement of Hip Joint Motion during Walking, Evaluation of an Electrogoniometric Method, J. Bone Jnt. Surg., 51A, 1083, 1969.

32. Lamoreux, L.W. Kinematic Measurements in the Study of Human Walking, Bulletin of Prosthetic Research, BPR-10-15, 3, 1971.

33. Townsend, M.A., Izak, M. and Jackson, R.W., Total Motion Knee Goniometry, J. Biomechanics, 10, 183, 1977.

34. Kinzel, G.L., Hillberry, B.M., Hall, A.S., Jr., Van Sickle, D.C., and Harvey, W.M., Measurement of the Total Motion between Two Body Segments--II, Description of Application, J. Biomechanics, 5, 283, 1972.

35. Morris, J.R.W., Accelerometry - A Technique for the Measurement of Human Body Movements, J. Biomechanics, 6, 729, 1973.

36. Light, L.H., McLellan, G. and Klenerman, L., Skeletal Transients on Hell Strike in Normal Walking with Different Footwear, J. Biomechanics, 13, 477, 1980.

37. Dempster, W.T., Space Requirements of the Seated Operator, WADC Technical Report, Wright-Patterson AFB, Ohio, 55, 1955.

38. Clauser, C.E., McConville, and Young, J.T., Weight, Volume and Centre of Mass of Segments of the Human Body. Report No. AMRL-TR-69-70, Wright-Patterson AFB, Ohio, 1969.

39. Chandler, R.F., Clauser, C.E., McConville, J.T., Reynolds, H.M. and Young, J.W., Investigation of Inertial Properties of the Human Body, Report No. AMRL-TR-74-137, Wright-Patterson AFB, Ohio, 1975.

40. Liu, Y.K. and Wickstrom, J.K., Estimation of the Inertial Property Distribution of the Human Torso from Segmented Cadaveric Data, Perspectives in Biomedical Engineering, Kenedi, R.M., Ed., MacMillan Press, London, 1973, 203-213.

41. Fisher, O., Der Gang des Menschen, Abh, Math. Phys. Cl. Kon. Sachs. Ges. Wissensch, II-25, 1900, 1, III-26, 1901, 85, IV-26, 1901, 469, V-28, 1904, 319, VI-28, 1904, 531.

42. Barter, J.T. Estimation of the Mass of Body Segments, WADC Technical Report 57-260, Wright-Patterson Air Force Base, Ohio, 1957.

43. Zatsiorsky, V. and Seluyanov, V., The Gamma Mass Scanning Technique for Inertial Anthropometric Measurement, J. Biomechanics (in press).

44. Drillis, R.J. and Contini, R., Body Segment Parameters, Technical Report No. 1166.03, School of Engineering and Science, New York Univ., 1966.

45. Hanavan, E.P., A Mathematical Model of the Human Body, Report No. AMRL-TR-102, Wright-Patterson AFB, Ohio, 1964.

46. Jensen, R.K., Estimation of the Biomechanical Properties of Three Body Types Using a Photogrammetric Method, J. Biomechanics, 11, 349, 1978.

47. Hatze, H., A Mathematical Model for the Computational Determination of Parameter Values of Anthropomorphic Segments, J. Biomechanics, 13, 833, 1980.

48. Miller, D.J. and Morrison, W.E., Prediction of Segmental Parameters Using the Hanavan Human Body Model, Med. Sci. Sports, 7, 207, 1975.

49. Cappozzo, A, The Forces and Couples in the Human Trunk during Level Walking, J. Biomechanics, 16, 265, 1983.

50. Vaughan, C.L., Andrews, J.G. and Hay, J.G., Selection of Body Segment Parameters by Optimization Methods, J. Biomech. Engng., 104, 38, 1982.

51. Cappozzo, A., Leo, T. and Pedotti, A., A General Computing Method for the Analysis of Human Locomotion, J. Biomechanics, 8, 307, 1975.

52. Andrews, B. and Jones, D., A Note on the Differentiation of Human Kinematic Data, Dib. 11th Internat. Conf. on Medical and Biological Engng. Ottawa, 88, 1976.

53. Lanshammar, H., On Practical Evaluation of Differentiation Techniques for Human Gait Analysis, J. Biomechanics, 15, 99, 1982.

54. Cappozzo, A., Leo, T. and Macellari, V., The CoSTEL Kinematics Monitoring System: Performance and Use in Human Movement Measurements, Biomechanics VIII-A., Matsui, H., and Kobayashi, K., Eds., Human Kinetics Pub, Champaign, 1982.

55. Plagenhoef, S.C., Computer Programs for Obtaining Kinetic Data on Human Movements, J. Biomechanics, 1, 221, 1968.

56. Dierckx, P., An Algorithm for Smoothing, Differentiation and Integration of Experimental Data Using Spline Functions, J. Comp. Appl. Nat., 1, 165, 1975.

57. Wood, G.A. and Jennings, L.S., On the Use of Spline Functions for Data Smoothing, J. Biomechanics, 12, 477, 1979.

58. Jackson, M.K., Fitting of Mathematical Functions to Biomechanical Data, IEEE Trans., Biomed. Eng., BME-26 2, 122, 1979.

59. Winter, D.A., Sidwall, H.G. and Hobson, D.A., Measurements and Reduction of Noise in Kinematics of Locomotion, J. Biomechanics, 7, 157, 1974.

60. Gustafsson, L. and Lanshammar, H., ENOCH An Integrated System for Measurement and Analysis of Human Gait, Institute of Technology, Uppsala University, S-751-21, Uppsala, Sweden, 1977.

61. Lesh, M.D., Mansour, J.M. and Simon, S.R., A Gait Analysis Subsystem for Smoothing and Differentiation of Human Motion Data, J. Biomech. Eng., Trans. ASME, 101, 205, 1979.

62. McClellan, J.H., Parks, T.W., and Rabiner, L.R., A Computer Program for Designing Optimum FIR Linear Phase Filters, Audio Electroac, IEEE Tran. AU-21, 506, 1973.

63. Andrews, B., Cappozzo, A. and Gazzani, F., A Quantitative Method for Assessment of Differentiation Techniques Used for Locomotion Analysis, Computing in Medicine, Paul, J.P., Ferguson-Pell, M.W., Jordan, M.M., and Andrews, B.J., Eds, The MacMillan Press, London, 146, 1982.

64. Hamming, R.W., Digital Filters, Englewood Cliffs, Prentics Hall, 1977.

65. Anderssen, R.S. and Bloomfield, P., Numerical Differentiation Procedures for Non-Exact Data, Numer. Math., 22, 157, 1974.

66. Hatze, H., The Use of Optimally Regularized Fourier Series for Estinating Higher-Order Derivatives of Noisy Biomechanical Data, J. Biomechanics, 14, 13, 1981.

67. An, K.N., Hui, F.C., Morrey, B.F., Linscheid, R., and Chao, E. Muscles Across the Elbow Joint: A Biomechanical Analysis, J. Biomechanics, 14, 659, 1981.

68. Morrison, J.B. The Forces Transmitted by the Human Knee Joint During Activity, Ph.D. Dissertation, University of Strathclyde, Glasgow, 1967.

69. Morrison, J.B., Bioengineering Analysis of Force Actions Transmitted by the Knee Joint, Biomed. Eng., 4, 164, 1968.

70. Paul, J.P., Bio-Engineering Studies of the Forces Transmitted by Joints: I. Engineering Analysis, Biomechanics and Related Bio-Engineering Topics, Kenedi, R.M., Ed., Pergamon Press, Oxford, 1965, 369.

71. Paul, J.P., Forces Transmitted by Joints in the Human Body, Proc. Inst. Mech. Eng. 3J, 1967, 181.

72. Paul, J.P., and Poulson, J., The Analysis of Forces Transmitted by Joints in the Human Body, Proc. Int. Conf. Exper, Stress Anal., Udine, Italy, 1974.

73. Heydinger, G.J., Upper Limb Joint External Force and Moment Determination and Resultant Elbow Joint Force Prediction, Masters Thesis, Ohio State University, Columbus, 1985.

74. Toft, R. and Berme, N. A Biomechanical Analysis of the Joints of the Thumb, J. Biomechanics, 13, 353, 1980.

75. Berme, N., Nicol, A.C., and Pual, J.P. A Biomechanical Analysis of Elbow Joint Function, I. Mech. Eng., 46, 1977.

76. Berme, N., Paul, J., and Purves, W, Biomedical Analysis of the Metacarpophalangeal Joint, J. Biomechanics, 10, 405, 1977.

77. Cnockaert, J.C., Lensel, G. and Pertuzon, E., Relative Contribution of Individual Muscles to the Isometric Contraction of a Muscle Group, J. Biomechanics, 8, 387, 1975.

78. Chao, E.Y., Apgrande, J.O., and Axmear, F.E., Three-Dimensional Force Analysis of Finger Joints in Selected Isometric Hand Functions, J. Biomechanics, 9, 387, 1976.

79. An, K.N., Kwak, B.M., Chao, E.Y., and Morrey, B.F., Determination of Muscle and Joint Forces: A New Technique to Solve the Indeterminate Problem, Transactions of the ASME 106, 364, 1984.

80. Basmajian, J.V. and Latif, A, Integrated Actions and Functions of Chief Flexors of the Elbow, J. Bone Jt. Surg., 39-A, 1957.

81. Stormont, T.J., An, K.N, Morrey, B.F., and Chao, E.Y., Elbow Joint Contact Study: Comparison of Techniques, J. Biomechanics, 18, 329, 1985.

82. Pauwels, F. Biomechanics of the Locomotor Apparatus, Springer-Verlag, Heidelberg, New York, 1980.

83. Amis, A.A., Dowson, D., and Wright, V., Elbow Joint Force Predictions for Some Strenuous Isometric Actions, J. Biomechanics, 13, 765, 1980.

84. Hui, F.C., Chao, E.Y., and An, K.N., Muscle of Joint Forces at the Elbow Joint During Isometric Lifting, Transactions of the 24th Annual Meeting of Orthopaedic Research Society, 3, 167, 1978.

85. Ikai, M. and Fukunaga, T.R., Calculation of Muscle Strength Per Unit Cross-Sectional Area of Human Muscle by Means of Ultrasonci Measurements, Int. Z. Angewandte Physiol, 26, 26, 1968.

86. Simpson, D., An Examination of the Design of an Endoprochesis for the Elbow, M.Sc. Thesis, University of Strathclyde, Glasgow 1975.

87. Nicol, A.C., Berme, N., and Paul, J.P., A Biomechanical Analysis of Elbow Joint Function, I. Mech. Engr., 45, 1977.

88. Bankov, S., and Jorgensen, K., Maximum Strength of Elbow Flexors with Pronated and Supinated Forearm, Communications from the Danish National Association for Infantile Paralysis, 29, 1969.

89. Penrod, D.D., Davy, D.T., and Singh, D.P., An Optimization Approach to Tendon Force Analysis, J. Biomechanics, 7, 123, 1974.

90. Yeo, B.P., Investigations Concerning the Principle of Minimal Total Muscular Force, J. Biomechanics, 9, 413, 1976.

91. Seireg, A. and Arvikar, R.J., The Prediction of Musclar Load Sharing and Joint Forces in the Lower Extremities During Walking, J. Biomechanics, 8, 89, 1975.

92. Hardt, D.E., Determining Muscle Forces in the Leg During Normal Human Walking - An Application and Evaluation of Optimization Methods, Transactions of the ASME 100, 72, 1978.

93. Chao, E.Y. and An, K.N., Determination of Internal Forces in Human Hand, J. Eng. Mech. Div., 104, 255, 1978.

94. Crowninshield, R.D., Use of Optimization Techniques to Predict Muscle Forces, Transactions of the ASME 100, 88, 1978.

95. Pedotti, A., Krishnan, V.V., and Stark, L., Optimization of Muscle-Force Sequencing in Human Locomotion, Math. Bio. 38, 57, 1978.

96. Patriarco, A.G., Mann, R.W., Simon, S.R., and Mansour, J.M., An Evaluation of the Approaches of Optimization Models in the Prediction of Muscle Forces During Human Gait, J. Biomechanics, 14, 513, 1981.

97. Crowninshield, R.D. and Brand, R.A., A Physiologically Based Criterion of Muscle Force Prediction in Locomotion, J. Biomechanics, 14, 793, 1981.

98. Fick, R., Handbuck der Anatomic des Menschen, Gustav Fischer Vol. 2, 1910.

99. Dons, B., Bollerup, K., Bonde Peterson, F., and Hancke, S. The Effect of Weight-lifting Exercise Related to Muscle Fiber Composition and Muscle Cross-sectional Area in Humans, Eur. J. Appl. Physiol., 40, 95, 1979.

100. Cope. R. An Optimization Approach to the Understanding of Time-Varying Leg-Muscle Froces, Ph.D. Dissertation, Ohio State University, Columbus, Ohio, 1986.

THE TENSION-LENGTH AND FORCE-VELOCITY RELATIONSHIPS
OF HUMAN MUSCLE IN SITU

S. Bouisset
Université de Paris-Sud, Orsay, France

The title of this lecture covers a twofold interrogation: i) are the mechanical properties of the human muscle the same as those described for animals? ii) do the conditions of muscle contraction during natural motor activity allow these properties to be apparent in any situation? These questions will be examined in relation to the characteristic relations, i-e tension-length and force-velocity curves, which defines the mechanical behavior of the generator of muscular force.*

*A preliminary report on this topic was given at the VIIth International Congress of Biomechanics held at Warzawa in 1979 (Bouisset, 1982).

I- MECHANICAL PROPERTIES OF MUSCLE.

A. Characteristic relations in the isolated muscle.

The   fundamental property of a muscle is its response to a
stimulation by a contraction i.e., a succession of internal processes
whose external result is the development of a force which tends to bring
the muscle's origin and insertion closer together.

Experimental conditions.

The   isolated muscle is studied under precise conditions: i)
conditions of stimulation: synchronous stimulation of all the muscular
fibers is used. More precisely, it is in most cases a maximal
stimulation since it is much easier to examine the mechanical state of
the active muscle in the stationary state of the tetanus than in the
transient state of the twitch; ii) mechanical conditions: two situations
are studied, the one where the length of the muscle is maintained
constant (isometric conditions) and the other where the tension remains
constant while the length varies (anisometric isotonic conditions). In
all cases the mechanical variables of the contraction are measured at
the tendon in the direction of the line of action of the muscle.

Characteristic relations.

A characteristic relation corresponds to each mechanical condition.

Isometric   conditions: tension-length curve. The muscle is
maintained at a given length. If it is tetanized, the muscle responds by
developing a tension. If it is brought to different lengths prior to the

stimulation, the tension appears to be a function of the length.

The relationship between isometric tension and length presents a sigmoïd shape, now classic, of which the point of inflexion corresponds approximately to the resting length.

Isotonic conditions: force-velocity curve. The muscle is free to change its length. If it is tetanized, it displaces the load which is applied to it as soon as its tension is sufficient. From this instant the tension and the shortening velocity of the muscle remain constant. The greater the load, the lower the shortening velocity: maximum for zero load, the velocity is zero when the load corresponds to the maximal isometric tension.

The relationship between the isotonic force and the shortening velocity can be fitted by different curves. The hyperbolic fitting (Hill, 1938) is certainly the most well known. It should be noted that when the shortening of the muscle occurs, starting from an initial length which is different from the resting length (Abbott and Wilkie, 1953), the diminution of the isometric tension should be taken into account.

Furthermore, if one applies to the muscle in contraction loads superior to its maximal isometric tension, it lengthens at a constant velocity. So a simple relationship as before between load and velocity is no longer observed (Aubert, 1956).

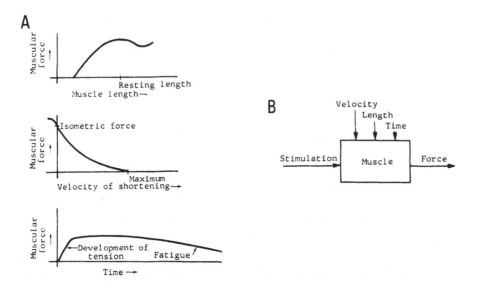

Fig.1 The muscle, considered as a force generator. A-Dependence of muscular force on variable other than electrical stimulation, i.e., the three internal non-linearities of the muscle (from top to bottom: force-length, force-velocity and force-time curves). B-Symbolic representation of the muscle with its nonlinearities: to know the stimulation level is not sufficient to determine the value of muscular force, (modified from Houk and Henneman, 1968).

These characteristic relations show an obvious generality in the sense that their general shape, i.e., their equation is the same for all muscles, and all fibers, of vertebrates studied until now. On the other hand, their parameters of shape, i.e., the coefficients of their equation, vary from one muscle to another for the same animal and from one species to another. These physiological differences are a consequence of the morphological and structural diversity of the muscles. Because of this, the particular properties of a muscle in Man are difficult to extrapolate from data established in animals.

Interpretations.

From a mechanical point of view, a muscle can be represented as a contractile component in series with an elastic component and in parallel to another elastic one. This identification is problably an oversimplification but is very useful in understanding the mechanical behavior of a muscle.

From a system analysis point of view, it should be pointed out that the muscle is not an ideal generator of force (Houk and Henneman, 1968). That is to say, for a given constant level of excitation, the tension developed by a muscle depends on the conditions of the contraction and in particular on the mechanical conditions under which it is performed. The effect of the time factor constitutes a supplementary non-linearity (see Fig.1).

B. Characteristic relations in the normal human muscle.

The study of mechanical properties of human normal muscle can only be done on muscle in the body since one cannot take as representative those studies carried out on muscles of amputees (Ralston et al, 1949).

As is known, the elementary movement is mono-articular, and the measurements are done at the periphery of the body. As compared to the study of the isolated muscle, that of the muscle in situ is complicated in particular by the fact that: i) the quantities measured are transformed by the geometry of the musculo-skeletal system; and ii) the quantities measured result from the contraction of a muscle group rather from that of a single muscle (see Fig.2).

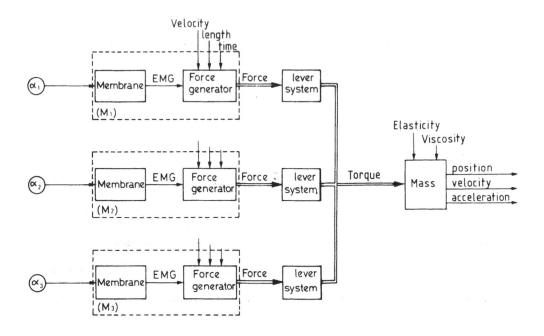

<u>Fig.2</u> Schematic representation of a muscle group in situ. The muscle group which is considered includes three agonist muscles (M_1, M_2, M_3). Each muscle (represented by a dashed box) is divided into a membrane and a force generator: each fiber membrane is depolarized, as a consequence of an efferent signal (α motoneuron) and each elementary depolarization results in a global signal (EMG) which is an entry to the force generator. The output of each muscle, when contracting, is a force which tends to bring its origin and insertion closer together. The force exerted by each muscle is transformed by the lever system into a torque which is applied to a mass located at body periphery level. The torque may result in a displacement of the mass, which could be modified by external elasticities and viscosities. The force developed by each of the three agonist muscles is applied to the same mass through different musculo-skeletal geometry, i.e., transformed by different lever systems. Mechanical connections are shown with double lines

Experimental conditions.

The human muscle in situ should be studied in a preparation which fulfills certain precise criteria well defined by Wilkie (1950): a joint having a simple musculo-skeletal geometry and a mono-articulated movement. These criteria are substantially satisfied by very few movements. This is the case of the elbow flexion on which most studies have been carried out.

In order to allow comparisons, conditions are used that approach as closely as possible the study of the isolated muscle. In so doing, two types of consequences are encountered: i) conditions of stimulation: subjects are asked to exert a maximal effort which in turn produces the most favorable situation to obtain conditions of constant stimulation, even if they are not necessarily maximal. However, the excitation of muscular fibers cannot be considered synchronous, which is a different from the isolated muscle; ii) mechanical conditions: the use of an ergometer allows these conditions to be fixed; for example, the position of the joint at a predetermined angle and the applicaton of either static or dynamic external torques. Thus the muscular group is placed in a situation of isometric or anisometric contractions. Insofar as the isotonic conditions are concerned, the muscular force must be constant requiring here not only that the applied force and velocity of movement be constant but also that the effect of angular variations be negligible.

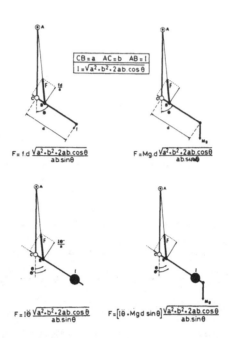

$$F = f.d \frac{\sqrt{a^2+b^2+2ab.\cos\theta}}{ab.\sin\theta} \qquad F = Mg.d \frac{\sqrt{a^2+b^2+2ab.\cos\theta}}{ab.\sin\theta}$$

$$F = I\ddot{\theta} \frac{\sqrt{a^2+b^2+2ab.\cos\theta}}{ab.\sin\theta} \qquad F = [I\ddot{\theta} + Mgd\sin\theta] \frac{\sqrt{a^2+b^2+2ab.\cos\theta}}{ab.\sin\theta}$$

Fig.3 Calculation of the force of biceps, the flexor muscle equivalent. The force F, developed by the muscle equivalent, is calculated under four conditions: Upper row: isometric contraction exerted against a resistance, f, which is perpendicular to the direction of the forearm (left side), and against a load, Mg (right side). Lower row: anisometric contraction exerted against a pure inertia, I (left side) and against inertia, I and a load, Mg (right side). The significance of symbols, a, b, and I, the length of the muscle equivalent, is indicated in the insert. The angle of the forearm is measured with relevance to its position in full extension. It can be noticed that in the condition of a movement, the force, F, can be constant, i.e., the contraction can be called isotonic, only if does not vary too much. Moreover, for movements performed against an inertia and a load, the acceleration has to be small or null, i.e., the velocity has to be constant; for movements performed against a pure inertia, isotonic conditions require that the acceleration be constant, a condition which can only be fulfilled approximately in slow movements.

Characteristic relations.

In order to trace the characteristic relations, it is necessary to have available appropriate linear quantities. However, the articular movement only produces angular cinematic variables and torques.
The linearization of these data can be realized either directly by technical means or indirectly by electronic or computer ones. Because of this, it is necessary to choose a point and a direction of measurement: either the wrist or the insertion of the biceps (for the elbow flexion) and the line of action of the biceps or a direction close to it. When all the quantities are related to one muscle of the group, the biceps for example, it is, in a way, as if this muscle is considered as representative of the whole. Such a muscle can be named a "Muscle equivalent", (Fig.3), and the hypotheses under which this representativity is effective have been defined (Bouisset, 1973).

In all cases the external force which is registered is actually the resultant of the forces exerted by each of the elbow flexors. On the other hand, the velocity and the length are actually those of the point of measurement according to the direction considered.

It is based on these quantities that the characteristic relations of the in situ muscle are studied. These relations present the same shape as those established for the isolated muscle in comparable experimental conditions.

Isometric conditions: by associating to each value of the length of the biceps the corresponding isometric force, Pertuzon (1972) found a tension-length relation with a sigmoid shape.

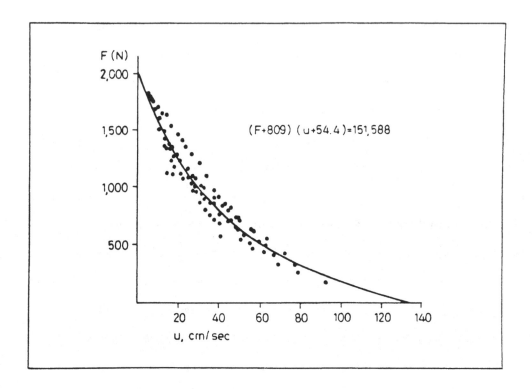

Fig.4 Instantaneous force—velocity relation in maximal movement. The points correspond to six maximal movements performed against various inertia (from 0,1 to 1,118 kg, m^2) by one individual. The curve in fitted by the equation shown in the figure. Forces, F, and velocities, u, are calculated for biceps, considered as muscle equivalent. This relation is only valid during the time interval when the level of excitation of each flexor muscle, based on the EMG, is approximately constant (and of their antagonists remains negligible), which is not the case, for example, at the beginning of the movement, (from Pertuzon and Bouisset, 1972).

Anisometric conditions: two sub-modalities are considered and for each one the existence of the force-velocity relation in established: i) under isotonic conditions, where each value of the load is associated with the peak value of the velocity of the corresponding movement (Wilkie, 1950). The parameters of the relation vary according to the subject and even for the same subject depending on his degree of conditioning (Asmussen, 1973). A preliminary stretching of the muscle in contraction increases the value of its force for same shortening velocity (Cavagna et al, 1968). Moreover as for an isolated muscle, if the muscle is made to lengthen at a constant velocity, the simple relation between force and velocity is no longer observed (Komi, 1973). ii) Under anisotonic conditions, i.e., in the course of the same movement, where instantaneous values of the shortening velocity of the biceps and that of the corresponding force are associated, as shown in Fig.4 (Pertuzon and Bouisset, 1971). This relation has also been shown for the triceps (Cnockaert, 1976).

Interpretation in terms of single muscle.

The characteristic relations described can be accounted for as a property of the muscles themselves insofar as the level of excitation of all flexor muscles, based on the EMG, is approximately constant during the course of the motor activity (and that of their antagonists remains negligible).

Given this condition, it can be assumed that the human muscles follow tension-length and force-velocity curves, of which only the parameters vary from one muscle to another. Thus the properties found

experimentally   should   result   from   the   sum   of   the   characteristic
relations of each of the flexor muscles.

Among   the   various   indirect   arguments which support this opinion a
few   can   be   mentioned: i)   the   existence   of the individual relations
torque-angle   (Morecki   et   al,   1968) and force-velocity (Wilkie, 1950),
deduced   from   experimental   data   under   diverse   and in fact relatively
large   hypotheses;   and ii) the properties of the contractile and elastic
components   of   the   mscle,   such   as were described in particular on the
Muscle   Equivalent   (Pertuzon, 1972; Goubel, 1974; Cnockaert, 1976) which
are compatible with those described for the isolated muscle.

II   MECHANICAL   PROPERTIES   OF   THE   MUSCLE   AND   NATURAL   CONDITIONS OF
CONTRACTION.

The   muscle   is   often   contracted under conditions far removed from
those   under   which   the characteristic relations have been demonstrated.
Indeed   i)   the   excitation   of   the muscle is usually sub-maximal, often
instantaneously   variable,   and   cannot   be   considered   as   synchronous.
Moreover,   the   simultaneous   activity of other muscles may facilitate or
inhibit   that of the group studied; ii) external forces of various nature
and   instantaneously   variable   can   cumulate their mechanical effects on
the   muscle   so   that it is not necessarily placed in purely isometric or
isotonic conditions during the course of its contraction.

The   study   of   the mechnical properties of the muscle thus leads to
the   study,   as   before,   of   a mono-articulated movement and to place it
under   comparable   mechanical   conditions.   On the other hand, due to the

fact that the contraction is sub-maximal, the level of excitation of the muscle must be measured. Finally, relations are to be considered between two out of three quantities (level of excitation, force, length or velocity), the third one being kept constant.

A. Level of excitation of the muscle.

The level of excitation of the muscle is measured from the global EMG; that is to say, complex traces obtained by detection either from surface electrodes or from wire electrodes of low selectivity.

The discussion on this subject will be restricted to the following considerations: i) the global EMG well represents the level of excitation of the muscle insofar as it is related to the number and the discharge frequency of active MUs. The morphology of this EMG necessarily differs from that of an interferential recording of MU's, and even more from that of an elementary recording; ii) the surface EMG is a measure of the intra-muscular EMG (Maton et al, 1969; Bouisset and Maton, 1972); iii) the quantification of the level of excitation is normally realized by different techniques of integration of the EMG signal (see Bouisset, 1973). These consist either of a "true integration" (iEMG) —which is a quantity of electricity— or of an "envelope" which is either the continuous mean value or averaged EMG (Avg EMG) or the effective value (r.m.s.) of the EMG signal.

B. Characteristic relations and constant level of excitation.

The level of excitation is in general considered to be constant when the EMG fluctuates in a random fashion around a stable value. This condition does not imply necessarily a state of tetanus.

Isometric conditions.

It is now well established that: i) for a given articular angle the integrated EMG increases with the external force, most likely in a curvilinear fashion (see review by Bouisset, 1973); ii) a family of curves corresponds to different values of the angle (Vredenbregt and Koster, 1956).

If the relation (i) is only an expression of the mechanisms of the gradation of the force, the relations (ii) also result from the mechanical properies of the muscle. Indeed, a family of tension-length curves has been traced for different constant levels of iEMG (Pertuzon, 1972). It can be affirmed that it is in fact a muscular property since the level of excitation of the different muscles of the group increases in the same manner as a function of force (Maton and Bouisset, 1977).

Anisometric conditions.

In the case of movements of short amplitude for which external force and velocity are approximately constant, it has been shown that: i) for a given velocity the iEMG varies in a linear fashion with the force (Bigland and Lippold, 1954). The slope of the relationship is lower in the case of eccentric contractions. ii) for a given force the iEMG varies with the velocity in a linear fashion (Bigland and Lippold, 1954) or in a curvilinear way when a larger range of velocities is considered (Zahalak et al, 1976). The slope of the relationship is almost null when the muscle contracts during lengthening; iii) the iEMG varies in a linear way with the external work (Scherrer et al, 1957).

As above, the validity of the force-velocity relation in the case of submaximal contractions has to be assumed to be able to give a satisfactory explanation for both the relations (i) and (ii).
This result was directly demonstrated by Bigland and Lippold (1954) when they found a family of force-velocity curves corresponding to different levels of iEMG.

C. Characteristic relations and variable level of excitation.

This experimental situation which poses numerous difficulties has only been studied in a few particular cases.

"Isometric" conditions.

It has been shown that for a given articular angle the instantaneous Avg EMG increases in a curvilinear fashion with corresponding values of the tension (Zuniga and Simons, 1969). This result generalizes that established for stable levels of excitation in the case of steadily increasing isometric contractions.

Furthermore, if one admits that a movement performed at an extremely slow speed is similar to a succession of static contractions, the results of Bottomley et al. (1963) state that for a given value of the external force the Avg EMG varies with the articular angle in a manner which is not incompatible with the tension-length relation.

Anisometric conditions.

The only studies carried out in this case were done on movements performed against pure inertia. During these movements not only the EMG but also the force and the velocity vary at each instant. Considering the EMG integrated during the entire contraction of the muscle, the existence of relations between this index and diverse biomechanical quantities has been demonstrated (see review of Bouisset, 1973). These relations include: i) a linear relationship with the peak acceleration of the movement the slope of which depends on the inertia, and a linear relationship with the peak force which does not depend on the inertia; ii) a quadratic relationship with the peak velocity, the coefficients of which depend on inertia; iii) a linear relationship with the mechnical work. This relationship is the most pertinent insofar as it does not depend on either the inertia or the rate of excitation (Bouisset and Goubel, 1973). Moreover, its slope is steeper for concentric than for eccentric contractions (Cnockaert, 1976) and also depends on the starting angular position. Lastly, these relations hold true for each of the elbow flexors (Bouisset et al, 1977).

As above, these relations are likely to meet a twofold interpretation. Insofar as the characteristic curves are considered, it is important to point out that there is not relation between force and velocity. But from (ii), it is possible to find a family of curvilinear relationships between the peak velocity and inertia corresponding to different values of iEMG. It has been demonstrated that this inertia-velocity curve results from the mathematical transformation of the force-velocity curve in the case of contractions against pure inertia (Goubel, 1974). Moreover, the influence of the starting position which is valid for each relation, even though it was just described for relation (iii), is a consequence of the tension-length relation.

On the other hand, insofar as it is known, neither relations between instantaneous values of biomechanical quantities nor between certain of these and the level of instantaneous excitation have been shown. The study of such relations first necessitates an appropriate index of the EMG. It also requires that the experimental conditions under which the characteristic relations are brought to light be respected. These conditions are, as has been seen, quite strict from a mechanical point of view in order to avoid, among other things, interference from the effects of length and velocity on the force. They are also strict concerning the level of excitation which must present a certain constancy so that the generator of force can effectively develop an isometric force of reference such as shown by Goubel (1974). As a consequence, it can be asked, if as soon as the level of excitation is instantaneously variable, it is realistic to hope to demonstrate the characteristic relations except under very particular conditions.

CONCLUSIONS.

i) With respect to the question of knowing if the mechanical properties of the human muscle are similar to those described for animals, the reply is positive. Indeed, the validity of the relations tension-length and force-velocity for man can be accepted.

ii) With respect to the question of knowing if the conditions of muscle contraction during natural motor activities allow these relations to be derived in their canonical form under any circumstance, the answer must obviously be negative. As a matter of fact, these equations correspond to very limited conditions. During a given motor activity, the more the conditions of contraction depart from these limited conditions, the higher the probability that the relationships between the force and the length and/or the velocity differ from their simple original form. It should be a fortiori the case for pluri-articular movements.

iii) Consequently, if the surface EMG signal can be considered as an appropriate index for the level of muscle excitation, it seems rather hazardous to give it a simple mechanical significance in the case of complex motor activities.

REFERENCES

1. Bouisset, S., Mechanical properties of the human muscle involved in natural motor activities., Invited lecture, 7th Int. Congress of Biomechanics, Varzawa 1979, Biomechanics VII, Moreki, A. and Fidelus, K. Ed., Univ. Park Press, Penn. State, 1981, vol.B, 351-360.

2. Hill, A.V., The heat of shortening and the dynamic constants of muscle, Proc. Roy. Soc. B., 128, 263-274, 1938.

3. Abbott, B.C. and Wilkie, D.R., The relation between velocity of shortening and the tension-length curve of skeletal muscle, J. Physiol., London, 120, 214-223, 1953.

4. Aubert, X., Le couplage énergétique de la contraction musculaire, Arscia, Bruxelles, 1956, 315p.

5. Houk, J. and Henneman, E., Feedback control of movement and posture, in Medical Physiology, V.B. Mountcastle Ed., Mosby, St. Louis, 1968, 1581-1696.

6. Ralston, H.J., Polissar, M.J., Inman, V.T., CLose, J.R. and Feinstein, B., Dynamic features of human isolated voluntary muscle in isometric and free contractions, J. Appl. Physiol., 1, 526-533, 1949.

7. Wilkie, D.R., The relation between force and velocity in human muscle, J. Physiol., London, 110, 249-280, 1950.

8. Bouisset, S., EMG and force in normal motor activities, in New Developments in Electromyography and Clinical Neurology, J.E. DESMEDT, Ed., Karger, Basel, 1973, 547-583.

9. Pertuzon, E. La contraction musculaire dans le mouvement volontaire maximal, Ph. D. Thesis, Lille, 1972.

10. Asmussen, E., Growth in muscular strength and power, Physical Activity Human Growth and Development, Academic Press, New York, 1973, 59-79.

11. Cavagna, G., Dusman, B. and Margaria, R., Positive work done by a previously stretched muscle, J. Appl. Physiol., 24, 21-32, 1968.

12. Komi, P.V., Relationships between muscle length, muscle tension, EMG and velocity of contraction under eccentric and concentric contractions, in New Developments in Electromyography and Clinical Neurology, J.E. DESMEDT, Ed., Karger, Basel, 596-606, 1973.

13. Pertuzon, E. and Bouisset, S., Maximum velocity of movement and maximum velocity of muscle shortening, in Biomechanics II, Vredenbregt and Wartenweiller Eds., Karger, Basel, 1971, 170-173.

14. Cnockaert, J.C., Recherche des conditions optimales d'exécution de mouvements simple, à partir de critères biomécaniques et électromyographiques, Ph. D. Thesis, Lille, 1976.

15. Morecki, A., Ekiel, J., Fidelus, K. and Nazarczuk, K., Investigation of the reciprocal participation of muscles in the movements of the upper limbs of man, Biofizika, 13, 2, 306-312, 1968.

16. Goubel, F., Les propriétés mécaniques du muscle au cours du mouvement sous-maximal., Ph. D. Thesis, Lille, 1974.

17. Maton, B., Metral, S. and Bouisset, S., Comparaison des activités électromyographiques globale et élémentaire au cours de la contraction statique volontaire. Electromyography, 9, 311-323, 1969.

18. Bouisset, S. and Maton, B., The quantitative relation between surface and intramuscular electromyographic activities for voluntary movement., Amer. J. Phys. Med., 51, 8, 285-295, 1972.

19. Vredenbregt, J. and Koster, W.G., Some aspects of muscle mechanics in vivo, I.P.O. Ann. Progr. Rep., 1, 94-100, 1966.

20. Maton, B. and Bouisset, S., The distribution of activity among the muscles of a single group during isometric contraction, Europ. J. Appl. Physiol., 37, 101-109, 1977.

21. Bigland, B. and Lippold, O.C.J., The relation between force, velocity and integrated electrical activity in human muscles, J. Physiol., London, 123, 214-224, 1954.

22. Zahalak, G.I., Duffy, J., Stewart, P.A., Litchman, H.M., Hawley, R.H. and Paslay, P.R., Partially activated Human Skeletal Muscle: An experimental investigation of force, velocity and EMG., J. Appl. Mech., 98, 1, 81-86, 1976.

23. Scherrer, J., Bourguignon, A. and Marty, R., Evaluation électromyographique du travail statique, J. Physiol., Paris, 49, 376-378, 1957.

24. Zuniga, E.N. and Simons, D.G., Non linear relationship between averaged electromyogram potential and muscle tension in normal subsjects. Arch. Phys. Med., 50, 613-620, 1969.

25. Bottomley, A., Kinnier Wilson, A.B. and Nightingale, A., Muscle substitutes and myo-electric control., J. Brit. I.R.E., 439-448, 1963.

26. Bouisset, S. and Goubel, F., Integrated electromyographical activity and muscle work, J. Appl. Physiol., 35, 695–702, 1973.

27. Bouisset, S., Lestienne, F. and Maton, B., The stability of synergy in agonists during the execution of a simple voluntary movement. Electroenceph. Clin. Neurol., 42, 543–551, 1977.

ANALYSIS OF HUMAN LOCOMOTION
BY ADVANCED TECHNOLOGIES AND METHODOLOGIES

A. Pedotti, C. Frigo, R. Assente, G. Ferrigno
Politecnico di Milano, Milan, Italy

ABSTRACT

In recent years the more advanced gait analysis laboratories have been involved in developing instrumentation and methods for the assessment of walking performances.

Some of the new devices have been proposed for routinary clinical applications, but, in practice, despite a general interest demonstrated by clinicians operating in the areas of functional treatment, instrumental methods for gait analysis are rarely employed outside the research field.

At the Bioengineering Centre of Milan some new devices have been developed taking into account all the practical requirements for an easy and reliable application.

INTRODUCTION

Motor control, as well as other complex biological functions, for instance vision, are such common capabilities in animal Kingdom that we do not usually associate them with intelligence.

In common language we say that we are walking by foot or grasping by hand. We neglect that in both cases these are the result of a complex data processing performed by the brain, strictly integrated with other characteristic intellectual functions of man.

Very recently the foot prints testifying a bipedal walking of the australopitecus in a vulcanic desert in Tanzania, something like 375 millions of years ago, were discovered. This "biomechanical choice", allowing the freedom of upper limbs for skilled movements, is considered the beginning of a long process of evolution which charged both the brain and the way of locomotion, bringing finally to the man.

What is astonishing in this process is that we are, for the first time in our history, not only able to understand, at least to some extent, how we move but also to design and develop systems able to reproduce some of this complex functions. We refer to the new targets arising from the Artificial Intelligence and Robotics.

Therefore the analysis of human locomotion must be performed in the frame of the general knowledge of human being avoiding a pure mechanicistic approach.

Three points should be faced: what, how and why.

In the analysis of human locomotion "what" means those parts of the systems and the variables which must be considered first. (Pedotti.[1]).

Fig. 1 is a schematic representation of the systems involved in human locomotion control.

The CNS receives information on the external world by the visual, acustic and tactile systems and on the internal world by proprioceptors and vestibular system. The most important propioceptors involved in movement control are:

- the muscle spindles which provide the afferent pathways (from the periphery to the center) trains of spikes function of the muscle stretching and therefore considered transducers of muscle length;

- the Golgi organs located in the muscle tendons which are force transducers;

- the joint receptors which provide spikes function of the joint state and therefore considered transducers of joint angles;

- the vestibular system which gives information about the amplitude and direction of the head acceleration.

All these transducers are able to inform the CNS about the internal state of the system.

These data are processed by the CNS in a complex way and the result is a coordinated set of commands which, through the efferent pathways reach the muscular apparatus. How this complex data processing is performed, it is not completely clear yet, and constitutes one of the major problems still open in neurophysiology.

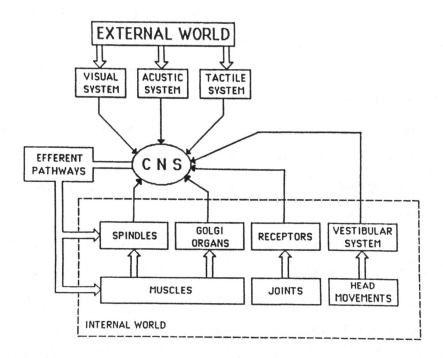

Figure 1 - Schematic representation of the systems involved in human locomotion control.

This knowledge can open new perspectives in the diagnosis of CNS lesions and can simultaneously provide new criteria for a better design of machines able to reproduce human functions, defining the characteristics of the second point we have cited above: "how".

Given the complexity of the biological system involved, the analysis of locomotion requires proper algorithms, and processing procedures strictly combined with specially designed apparata for detecting the meaning variables.

With this purpose at the Bioengineering Center of Milan special instrumentation has been developed which presents the following characteristics:

- reliability and accuracy in measurements;
- complete freedom of movement for the subject;
- on-line processing of the main data and presentation of results in a form easily understandable for the purpose of the analysis;
- real-time presentation of those variables which permit an immediate evaluation of the validity of the test.

In relation to the third point of this introduction the reasons why the analysis of human locomotion is performed should never be forgotten both in designing new algorithms or instrumentation and in defining testing procedures. Functional evaluation, rehabilitation diagnosis and therapeutic efficency control, which may be considered the main topics of human locomotion analysis, may require different testing procedures and specific computing on sets of variables, in accordance with the target of the analysis; flexibility of analysis systems, software and experimental set-up become, at this point, an extremely important variable to get proper results.

In the next paragraphs several systems, designed following the described criteria, are presented.

KINEMATICS MEASUREMENT

ELITE is a dedicated system designed and realized at the Bioengineering Center of Milan which is routinary used for automatic analysis of body movement in various conditions and environments.

Based on real-time processing of TV images, it recognizes multiple passive markers and computes their coordinates utilizing techniques derived directly from computer vision procedures, completely hardware implemented. (Ferrigno et al. [2], Ferrigno et al.[3]).

The system presents a two-level processing architecture, the first of which includes a dedicated peripheral fast processor for shape recognition, based on fast VLSI chips; the second level consists of a general purpose computer providing the overall system with high flexibility.

The points to be detected are marked on the subject by small hemispherical markers (diametre less than 7 mm) coated with reflective material; their weight is negligible at all and they can be easily fixed to the body by adhesive tape. The particular shape of the markers, makes them visible also when they rotate up to 60 degrees around their axes.

The main characteristic of ELITE system is the special algorithm which allows the recognition of markers only if their shape matches a predetermined "mask".

This is obtained in real time by a bidimensional cross-correlation of the TV image with a reference shape. All the pixels having a cross-correlation value above a prefixed threshold, and thus belonging to the image of a marker are extracted from the whole TV image. Thanks to the algorithm, the accuracy achieved by computing the centroid of a marker is up to 10 times the original one of the TV camera, reaching the value of one part in 2500 when standard analog TV cameras (256x256 pixels) are used. Moreover, ELITE system recognizes markers even in a noisy environment, including daylight, without restriction on the number of markers simultaneously detectable on the same frame.

The system actually works at 50 Hz sampling rate; preliminary results at 100 Hz have been obtained. The computer connected to the fast image processor provides for the following operations:

- data collection
- kinematic data enhancement (algorithm for increasing resolution, data reduction)
- 3D reconstruction (if more than one camera is used)
- calibration and distorsions correction
- modelling
- tracking of each marker and restoration of markers temporarily hidden by parts of the body during movement

- graphic representations

- data filtering

- velocities and accelerations computing.

Analysis of walking is in general performed by fixing markers on the iliac crest, the hip, the lateral femoral condyle, the lateral malleolus, the fifth metatarsal head and the heel. Figure 2 shows a stick diagram of a normal stride obtained by the above arrangement.

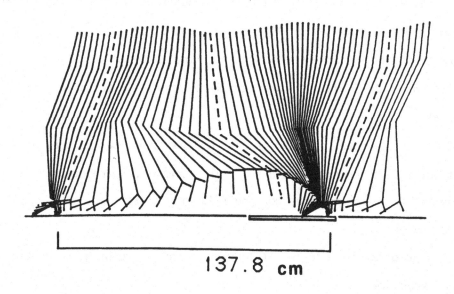

137.8 cm

Figure 2 - Stick diagram from a normal subject walking at his natural speed in front of a TV-camera. The elaboratioon is performed automatically by the ELITE system. Retroreflective markers are fixed on the iliac crest, the hip, the lateral femoral condile, the lateral malleolus, the fifth metatarsal head and the heel. Dashed lines correspond to heel strike and toe-off. Position of the force platform is reported. The lenght of the stride is reported below.

Modelling software procedures allow, in accordance with the
performed test, an automatic classification of the markers recognized on
each frame strictly reducing the time interval between consecutive
trials and allowing an on-line graphic representation of the data
acquired, useful to verify the correct execution of the test.

DYNAMICS MEASUREMENT

The use of a force-platform embedded into the floor in the middle of a pathway more than 16 m long was identified at the Bioengineering Center of Milan since 1975 as a primary tool for investigation of human locomotion, (Boccardi et al. [4]).

Vector diagram technique, consisting of a spatio-temporal representation of the ground reaction vectors produced while the foot is in contact with the floor, is a clinical oriented application providing highly meaningful results with high reliability and repeatibility beeing, at once, easy to use and little time consuming. (Rose. [5]).

The force is measured by a piezoelectric platform based on four quartz transducers installed one at each corner and sensitive to the 3 orthogonal components. The corresponding signals are acquired by an A/D converter connected to the host computer and displayed so as to represent the force vector in amplitude, direction and point of application. The sequence of the vectors projected on the sagittal plane describes a particular diagram (half-butterfly shaped, in normal walking) that is highly sensitive to alterations of gait. Dedicated software allows to compute different parameters, to compare data of patient referring to the same pathology and to analyze the evolution of the disease.

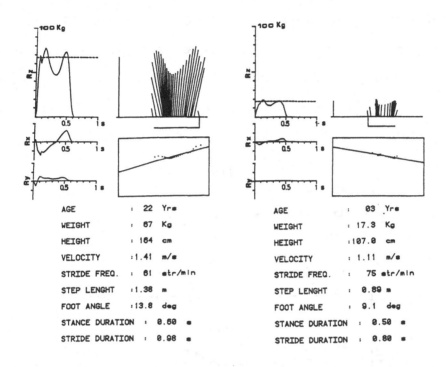

AGE	:	22 Yrs
WEIGHT	:	67 Kg
HEIGHT	:	164 cm
VELOCITY	:	1.41 m/s
STRIDE FREQ.	:	61 str/min
STEP LENGHT	:	1.38 m
FOOT ANGLE	:	13.8 deg
STANCE DURATION	:	0.60 s
STRIDE DURATION	:	0.98 s

AGE	:	03 Yrs
WEIGHT	:	17.3 Kg
HEIGHT	:	107.0 cm
VELOCITY	:	1.11 m/s
STRIDE FREQ.	:	75 str/min
STEP LENGHT	:	0.89 m
FOOT ANGLE	:	9.1 deg
STANCE DURATION	:	0.50 s
STRIDE DURATION	:	0.80 s

Figure 3 – Analysis of the ground reactions. On the left data from a normal subject 22 years old are reported, while on the right data refer to a normal child 3 years old. The time-course of the vertical (Rz), antero-posterior (Rx) and lateral (Ry) components are reported. Dashed line on the Rz graph represents the weight of the subject. The horizontal line corresponds to the distance between the anterior and posterior couple of transducers inside the force platform. The vertical line indicates the weight of the subject. A horizontal segment under the base line starts from the first vector and ends in correspondence with the last vector, indicating the direction of progression and the lenght of the support base. A top view of the force platform is reported under each vector diagram. The trajectory of the point of application of each vector (dots) has been fitted by a stright line obtained by means of a minimum square method in which a weight corresponding to the vertical component is given to each point. The angle of this regression line with the direction of progression has been called foot angle.

In Figure 3 a stride of an healthy adult subject on the left and the one of an healthy child on the right are reported.

By combining kinematics and dynamics data, contemporaneously acquired by the host computer, it is possible to compute the torques applied by the muscular groups at hip, knee and ankle joints during walking, adding more information to the analysis of the stride. (Boccardi et al. [6]). Figure 4 reports the time course of the joint torques obtained automatically during one stride of a patient.

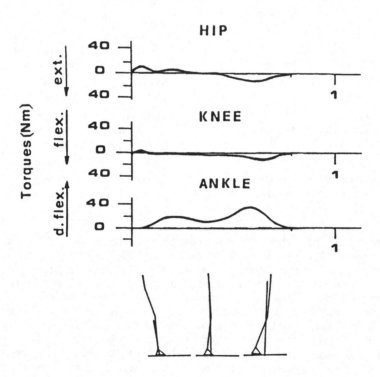

Figure 4 - Example of data elaboration: joint torques at hip, knee and ankle. On the lower part is a sequence of stick diagrams with the ground reaction vector superimposed. Each of them is approximately in correspondence with the time course of the above variables. This figure refers to a myodystrophic subject 9 years old not yet severely compromised.

SUPERIMPOSITION OF THE VECTOR TO THE TV IMAGE

For a direct approach to the analysis of the mechanical actions on
the joints due to the ground reaction a dedicated system has been
developed. It has been named DIGIVECT (digitized vector). (Ambrosini et al. [7]).

Figure 5 reports some examples of the possible applications.

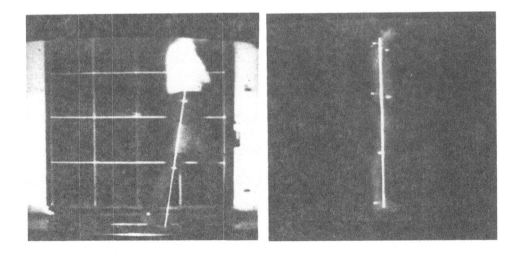

Figure 5 - Some of the possible uses of "DIGIVEC". The system allows
to superimpose on line the ground reaction vector   to   a TV-
image of the subject. On the left: gait analysis on the sagittal plane;
on the right: application to posture analysis.

Based on a Z80A microprocessor, it realizes a superimposition of the ground reaction vector to the image of the subject, providing significative results with simplified testing procedures applied not only to walking but also to the analysis of seated posture, for example, the action of loading one limb in subjects with impaired control of the load sharing mechanism, the analysis of scoliosis.

An use of this instrument as biofeedback system has been positively experimented too.

PODOBAR

When particular aspects of foot/floor or foot/shoes contact are to be investigated, such as the anomalies produced by orthopaedic pathologies of the foot or by peripheral vascular disease in diabetic patients, it is extremely important to know the distribution of load on different areas of the sole during walking.

PODOBAR is a system that answers this question. (Pedotti et al. [8], Assente et al. [9].).

A 200 um thick film of polyvinylidene fluoride (PVDF) has been uniaxially strectched up to a rate of 4:1 at a temperature of 85°C at a costant velocity of 0.8 cm/min; an annealing process has been perdormed by leaving the film between the jaws of the stretching machine at a temperature higher than 95°C for more than two hours. Sixteen circular sensors, 6 mm diametre each, have been obtained by poling the film at room temperature in silicon oil using a field of 2MV/cm applied for nearly 25 minutes in areas of the film arranged in order to match areas of the foot interesting for the analysis. The obtained film has been cut with insole shape and 16 conductive tracks have been deposited by vacuum evaporation of aluminium through a thin steel sheet, to bring electrical charges from each transducer to the connecting wires, which run along the patient's leg to an electronic unit fixed on it.

The electronic unit contains an analog multiplexer which sends in sequence the signal coming from each transducer to a charge amplifier which provide for signal conditioning in order to match properly the working range of the A/D converter of the host computer. The integration stage presents three different working modes depending on the configuration which is assumed by the multiplexer switch and another electronic switch connecting the operational amplifier to a reference voltage. The first working mode sets the integrator initial conditions by zeroing the integrator output. In the second mode the electronic switch is open and the multiplexer reads one of the 16 transducer channels allowing the integrator to process the charges coming from that specific transducer. When both the electronic and the multiplexer switches are open, the system is in hold and the value of the signal can be acquired by the computer. By proper synchronization of the three working modes, the output of all 16 transducers is read sequancially and repetitively.

The equipment provides also synchronizing signals to acquire data from each transducer of the insole at 100 Hz sampling rate

PVDF is sensitive to changes of the applied pressure and the electronic is designed to condition in sequence 16 different signals; for these reasons the data acquired quantify the variation of each signal every 10 ms. Software provides for the reconstruction of the pressure behaviour under the i-th transducers by integrating the acquired variations.

In figure 6 one of the more common distribution of the piezoelectric sensory areas and an example of localized pressure measurement during the supporting phase of a normal subject are reported.

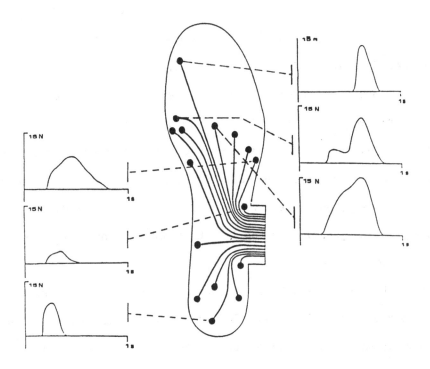

Figure 6 - PODOBAR - The arrangement of the sixteen piezoelectric transducers on the PVDF insole is presented. Signals provided by some of them are reported: fifth metatarsal head, lateral side, heel on the left side while big toe, first and second metatarsal head on the right.

OCTOPUS

It is an eight channel telemetric system for detection of the myoelectric activity. (Villa.[10]). It was designed in order to be the less encumbering as possible for the subject.

The portable equipment weights nearly 1 kg and includes preamplifiers, antialiasing filters, multiplexer, pulse duration modulation (PDM), transmitter and rechargeable batteries for power supply. It can be carried on the back and receives the wires from the electrodes. These last are commercially available bipolar surface electrodes that can be tied to the limb by elastic bands or glued to the skin (disposable version).

Four of the preamplifiers can be excluded by an external switching in order to allow auxiliary signals from particular devices, such as electrogoniometers or microswitches, to be transmitted as well. Figure 7 shows an integrated use of the above instrumentation.

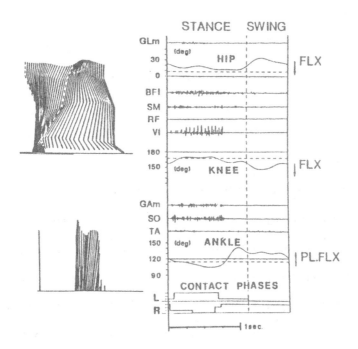

Figure 7 – Analysis of walking in a hemiplegic subject. On the left the stick and the vector diagrams are reported. On the right the joint angles (hip, knee and ankle) and the myoelectric activity of eight muscles detected during the same stride are presented (GLm = gluteus medius; BFe = biceps femoris caput longum; SM = semimembranosus; RF = rectus femoris; Vl = vastus lateralis; GAm = gastrocnemius medialis; So = soleus; TA = tibialis anterior). The two last graphs refer to the stride temporal phases of the two feet (L = left, R = right): first level = forefoot contact, second level = heel contact, third level = contact of the whole foot.

NEED FOR STANDARDIZATION

At present time a fruitful background has been prepared on the field of gait analysis by several investigations on human locomotion. (Cappozzo et al.[11], Pedotti [1], Boccardi et al.[12], Crenna and Frigo.[13]). Different technologically advanced systems for automatic gait analysis are already, or are going to become, commercially available and a wide spread of these new techniques in the fields of orthopaedics and functional rehabilitation is thus now available. In our opinion three phases can be singled out in which analytical measurements could be very useful:

1) assessment of residual walking capability. The analysis in this phase has two main purposes: a) to quantify parameters that could be used later-on as references to evaluate improvement; b) to single out the ·prime mechanisms causing a locomotory pattern and the compensating strategies;

2) individuation of the more appropriate intervention (tendon transportations, orthoses, functional electric stimulation) and

the parameters of such an intervention. In this phase the intervention can be evaluated by the effect on walking performance. In case of external aids or F.E.S. adaptation to the subject is thus possible;

3) monitoring medium and long term evolution of the pathology and evaluation of the effects of therapeutic interventions.

As described above the instrumentation available allow a rather complete analysis of walking to be performed. This doesn't mean that in every case the whole set up has to be employed. In our experience each different situation requires to consider the ratio between the resources employed (including the patient involvement) and the information gathered. For istance the first test session on a patient could require a wide analysis by means of the whole apparatus while the subsequent ones can be monitored by a sub-set of instrumentation (vector diagram, for example). In general the electromyographic analisis is the more time consuming one, mainly because of the time required for placing correctly the electrodes on the muscles. It can often be substituted, if the purely mechanical action at the joints is required, by the analysis of the joint torques obtainable by the Elite and force-platform systems. Personnels who work in the clinical field cannot be reasonably charged with the problem of setting up the more appropriate procedure but have to be facilitated in the choice by offering them some standardized solution particularly studied for the more common cases.

We can face the problem of standardization by considering first
what are the basic requirements for a gait analysis technique to be
used in clinics. In the opinion of R.A. Brand and R.D.
Crowninshield ([14]) : "....any patient evaluation tool will be useful
(and thus gain widespread acceptance) if, and only if, the technique
meets all the following criteria:

1) the measured parameter must correlate well with the patient's
   functional capability;

2) the measured parameter must not be directly observable and
   semiquantifiable by the physician or therapist (being able to add
   precision to a measurement does not necessary add to its value in
   the overall evaluation of the patient, particularly if the
   measurement is only one of many necessary in that evaluation);

3) the measured parameters must clearly distinguish between normal
   and abnormal;

4) the measurement technique must not significantly alter the
   performance of the evaluated activity;

5) the measurement must be accurated and reproducible;

6) the results must be communicated in a form which is readily identifiable in a physical or physiological analog.

This means that a first standardization in the procedure has to be achieved. Physicians who ask for a particular test of the gait have to be aware of the possibility to execute the test on that kind of pathology, they have to know which kind of information the method will furnish, the biomechanical significance of the variables analyzed and the limits of the procedure employed. Secondly even a well standardized procedure may furnish misleading results if different sign convention and scale for representation are used. Another important point is the reference to normal walking (barefooted or not, velocity ecc.), sex and age.

A clear definition of all these aspects, is imperative for every system worthy to be introduced in clinical practice. Standardization, if accepted and generalized, would enhance also the commercial possibility of introducing advanced instrumentations in the clinical field. Interchange of data between different laboratories would become easier and a useful background of knowledge would become available for improvement of treatments.

REFERENCES

1. Pedotti A., A study of motor coordination and neuromuscular activities in human locomotion, Biol. Cybernetics 26, 53, 1977.

2. Ferrigno G., Fogliani G., Frigo C., Pedotti A., ELITE: system for kinematic analysis of movement by real time processing of TV-signal, Proceedings of the IFAC-Inserm Workshop "Human Gait Analysis and Applications", Nov. 1983, Montpellier (France), P. Rabischong, A. Ligeois, E. Peruchon, Quick Print, Montpellier, 89, 1983.

3. Ferrigno G., Pedotti A., ELITE: a digital dedicated hardware system for movement analysis via real-time TV-signal processing, IEEE Trans, BME-32, 943, 1985.

4. Boccardi S., Chiesa G., Pedotti A., New procedure for evaluation of normal and abnormal gait, Am. J. Phys. Med. 56, 163, 1977.

5. Rose G.K., Clinical gait assessment: a personal view, J. of Med. Eng. and Technology, 7, 273, 1983.

6. Boccardi S., Pedotti A., Rodano R., Santambrogio G.C., Evaluation
    of muscular moments at the lower limb joints by an on-line
    processing of kinematic data and ground reaction, J. Biomech, 14,
    35, 1981.

7. Ambrosini A., Cometti A., Pedotti A., Santambrogio G.C., A new
    device for real-time analysis of posture and gait, Proceedings
    of the IFAC-Inserm Workshop "Human Gait Analysis and Applications",
    Nov. 1983, Montpellier (France), P. Rabishong, A. Ligeois and E.
    Peruchon, Quick Print, Montpellier, 77, 1985.

8. Pedotti A., Assente R., Fusi G., De Rossi D., Dario P., Domini-
    ci C., Multisensor piezoeletric polymer insole for podobarography,
    Ferroelectrics 60, 163, 1984.

9. Assente R., De Rossi D., Pedotti A., Rodano R., Piezoelectric
    multitransducer device to measure the dynamic loads beneath the
    foot, Proceedings of the IFAC-Inserm Workshop "Human Gait Analysis
    and Applications", Nov. 1983,Montpellier (France),P. Rabishong,
    A. Ligeois, and A. Peruchon, Quick Print, Montpellier, 39, 1985.

10. Villa A., Sistema biotelemetrico multicanale - Octopus -, Doctorial
    thesis, Politecnico di Milano, facolta' di Ingegneria, 1977.

11. Cappozzo A. Leo T., Pedotti A., A general computing method for the analysis of human locomotion, J. Biomech, Pergamon Press, 8, 307, 1975.

12. Boccardi S., Frigo C., Pedotti A., Tesio L., A biomechanical study of locomotion by hemiplegic patients, Biomech. VII, A. Morecki and K. Fidelus, Univ. Park Press, 1981.

13. Crenna P., Frigo C., Monitoring gait by a vector diagram technique in spastic patients, Restorative Neurology, vol. III, "Clinical Neurophysiology in Spasticity", P.J. Delwaide and R.R, Joung, Elsevier Science Publishers BV, 109, 1985.

14. Brand R.A., Crowninshield R.D., Comment on criteria for patient evaluation tools. Letters to the Editor, J. Biomech, 14, 9, 1980.

LIST OF LECTURERS

Berme Necip, Professor
 296, W. 18th Avenue
 Columbus, Ohio 43210
 USA

Bouisset Simon, Professor
 Lab. de Physiologie du Mouvement
 Université de Paris-Sud
 91405 Orsay
 France

Cappozzo Aurelio, Associate Professor
 Università degli Studi di Roma
 "La Sapienza"
 Ist. di Fisiologia Umana
 00100 Roma
 Italy

Komi Paavo, Professor
 Kinesiology Laboratory
 Dept. of Biology of Physical Activities
 University of Jyvaskyla
 SF - 40100 Jyvaskyla 10
 Finland

Morecki Adam, Professor
 Technical University of Warsaw
 Inst. for Aircraft Engineering and Applied Mechanics
 al. Niepodleglosci 222
 00-663 Warszawa
 Poland

Pedotti Antonio, Professor
 Centro di Bioingegneria
 Politecnico di Milano
 Fondazione Pro Juventute
 Via Gozzadini 7
 20148 Milano
 Italy

LIST OF PARTICIPANTS IN THE COURSE

Roberto ASSENTE, Researcher, Centro di Bioingegneria, Via Gozzadini 7 20148 Milano, Italy.

Francois BARRO, Doctor med., Dr.sc.math., Orthopädische Univ. Klinik Balgrist, Forchstrasse 8000 Zurich, Switzerland.

Giovanni CAMA, Medical Doctor, Istituto Superiore di Educazione Fisica di Roma, Viale Tito Livio 179, 00136 Roma, Italy.

Carlo CAPELLI, Medical Doctor, Via Tertulliano 48, 20137 Milano, Italy.

Federico CASOLO, Researcher, Politecnico di Milano, Dipartimento di Meccanica, Piazza Leonardo da Vinci 32, 20133 Milano, Italy.

Gurbuz CELEBI, Assoc. Professor, Ege University Medical School, Dept. of Basic Medical Sciences, Fizyoloji Anabilim Dali, Bornova, Izmir, Turkey.

Andrea CORVI, Researcher, Università di Firenze, Dip. di Meccanica e Tecnologie Industriali, Via S. Marta 3, 50139 Firenze, Italy.

Anna DABROWSKA, Research Assistant, Institute of Sport, ul. Ceglowska 68/70, 01-809 Warsaw, Poland.

Francesco DE BONA, Politecnico di Torino, Dipartimento di Meccanica, Corso Duca degli Abruzzi 24, 10129 Torino, Italy.

Hamed Ibrahim EL MOUSLY, Professor, Ain Shams University, Faculty of Engineering, Abbasiab, Cairo, Egypt.

Carlo FRIGO, Bioengineer Researcher, Centro di Bioingegneria, Politecnico di Milano, Via Gozzadini 7, 20148 Milano, Italy.

Jan GAJEWSKI, Research Assistant, Institute of Sport, ul. Ceglowska 68/70, 01-809 Warsaw, Poland.

Mary GARRET, Deputy Director, University College Dublin, School of Physiotherapy, 89 Fosters Avenue, Blackrock, co: Dublin, Ireland.

Hermann GREIFF, Assistant, University of Munster, FB20 Sportwissenschaft, Horstmarer-Londweg 62b, D-4400 Münster, West Germany.

Otmar KUGONIC, Ass. Professor, Fakulteta za Telesno Kulturo, Gortanova 22, 61000 Ljubljana, Yugoslavia.

Frank Friedbert LIEBSCHER, Assistant, Universität - Gesamthoschule Siegen, FB2 - Sportwissenschaft, Adolf-Reichweinstrasse, D-5900 Siegen, Wester Germany.

Vladimir MEDVED, Res. Assistant, University Zagreb, Faculty of Physical Culture, Horvacanski Zavoj 15, 41000 Zagreb, Yugoslavia.

Miroslaw NADER, Lecturer, Warsaw Technical University, Institute of Transport, ul. Koszykowsa 7, 00-662 Warsaw, Poland.

Wojciech NIWINSKI, Assistant, Warsaw Technical University, Nowowiejska 22/24, 00-665 Warsaw, Poland.

Fabio Massimo PEZZOLI, Doctor, Policlinico A. Gemelli, Largo A. Gemelli 8, 00168 Roma, Italy.

Renzo POZZO, Student, Via D. Moro 7, 33033 Codroipo (Udine), Italy.

Jean RIEU, Professor, Ecole des Mines, 42023 St. Etienne, France.

Paolo ROMANO, Ph.D. Bioengineer Student, DIST Università di Genova, Via Opera Pia 11a, 16145 Genova, Italy.i,

Raoul SAGGINI, Doctor, 1a Clinica Ortopedica, Via Tacca 20, Firenze, Italy.

Klaus-Peter SCHMOLL, Dipl. Math., Institut B of Mechanik, Universität Stuttgart, Pfaffenwaldring 9, D-700 Stuttgart 1, West Germany.

Hendrik VAN MAMEREN, Medical Doctor, Ryksuniversteit Limburg, Beeldonydersdreef 101, Maastricht, Holland.